The "30 Minute Change"

Learn to Change Anything In Your Life In 30 Minutes or Less!

Pat Sweeney

A PCS Services Inc. Publication

Published by:
PCS Services Inc.
Castaic Ca.

Library of Congress Control Number: 2017913873

ISBN-13:978-1975985004
1. Self Help 2. Human Behavior 3. Spirituality 4. Brain

Cover Design by Kelly Bloomfield
Printed in the United States of America
Author Contact: info@30MinuteChange.com

Additional Disclaimer:

The 30 Minute AOSED Change Process: The intent of the author is only to offer information of a general nature which can help you in your quest for emotional and spiritual well-being and thus the public must take complete responsibility for their use of it. Further, Pat Sweeney is not a licensed health professional and offers the information in this book solely as a life coach. Readers are strongly cautioned and advised to consult with a physician, psychologist, psychiatrist or other licensed health care professional before utilizing any of the information in this book. The information is based on information from sources believed to be accurate and reliable and every reasonable effort has been made to make the information as complete and accurate as possible but such completeness and accuracy cannot be guaranteed and is not guaranteed. The author, publisher, and contributors to this book, and their successors, assigns, licensees, employees, officers, directors, attorneys, agents and other parties related to them (a) do not make any representations, warranties or guarantees that any of the information will produce any particular medical, psychological, physical or emotional result, (b) are not engaged in the rendering of medical, psychological or other advice or services, (c) do not provide diagnosis, care, treatment or rehabilitation of any individual, and (d) do not necessarily share the views and opinions expressed in the information. If the reader purchases any services or products as a result of the information, the reader or user acknowledges that the reader or user has done so with informed consent. The information is provided on an "as is" basis without any warranties of any kind, express or implied. "The author, publisher, and contributors to this book, and their successors, assigns, licensees, employees, officers, directors, attorneys, agents and other parties related to them (a) expressly disclaim any liability for and shall not be liable for any loss or damage including but not limited to use of the information; (b) shall not be liable for any direct or indirect compensatory, special, incidental, or consequential damages or costs of any kind or character; (c) shall not be responsible for any acts or omissions by any party including but not limited to any party mentioned or included in the information or otherwise; (d) do not endorse or support any material or information from any party mentioned or included in the information or otherwise; (e) will not be liable for damages or costs resulting from any claim whatsoever. If the reader or user does not agree with any of the terms of the foregoing, the reader or user should not use the information in this book or read it. A reader who continues reading this book will be deemed to have accepted the provisions of this disclaimer.

*Special thanks to my oldest daughter
Michelle.
You have always believed in me and are
Instrumental in keeping me focused and
Faithful!*

CONTENTS

The Beginning..1

Chapter 1: Personal Growth 27

Chapter 2: Define and Find Your Dream Job...........................49

Chapter 3: Relationships...71

Chapter 4: New Hobbies..89

Chapter 5: Health & Fitness 101

Chapter 6: Finances 115

Chapter 7: Weight Control 127

Chapter 8: Parenting 139

The Ending 153

Appendix A: Whole-Brain Posture...159

References 161

The Beginning

*"It's not the wisest, strongest or most disciplined man who begins and ends
The journey. But I will tell you this. It will only be the man who, in spite of
His feelings, continues forward when darkness surrounds."*

The greatest journeys of all time began with a thought...followed by an action. The worst atrocities of this world also began with a thought... followed by an action. The most amazing humans born on this planet, of which you are one, began with a thought...followed by an action. Everything worthwhile you have ever done in your life began with a thought...followed by an action. And, unfortunately, everything you have wished you would have done, also began with a thought...followed by an action, of which the action was, to do nothing. Everyone has thoughts about a change they want to make, but very few have been trained in how to effectively turn those thoughts into New Beliefs which can then alter the course of one's life. I want to thank you for picking up a copy of this book and let you know that it was written with the belief that "if you build it, they will come." Or rather, "if I write it, they will read it."

I know that many of you want to make changes but have difficulty seeing them through. Some of you may really want to change but never seem to know how or where to start. Still

1

others of you may look at change as this ginormous mountain that you just can't climb anymore because you've tried before and every time you do, you fall back down and it adds another wound. Lastly, there are some of you who have a tendency to procrastinate or make excuses because "it's just too hard to change this in my life right now." I understand and have been there myself. There is a popular saying, "Give a person a fish, feed them for a day. Teach a person to fish, feed them for life." So I thought to myself: *Help a person change and they can hopefully make that one change. However, teach a person how to change and you can help them make changes for the rest of their life.* This was my inspiration for creating this New Change Process.

This book is going to teach you how to change anything in your life in "30 Minutes or Less". All I ask is that you sidebar your skepticism for a few hours. The techniques you will learn in this book, such as multi-sensory participation and Whole-Brain subconscious reprogramming, can be applied right away to make instant changes that will last. This process will help you to create and live out a New Belief about the change you want and give you the tools to implement that belief.

I always try to begin everything I do with the end in mind. As I began writing this book, the only questions I focused on were: What do I want you to believe after reading the book and what are the facts you need to know to do that? The answers: I want you to be inspired to believe and have a renewed internal confidence that you can and will make any change in your life, no matter how difficult, at any time you choose. All you need to do is take back your innate ability to not let the externals of the world affect the internal of who you were meant to be.

Before I clearly define the details of this "30 Minute Change" process that you will be using moving forward, I'd first like to share how I discovered and began implementing this in my own life.

I have bounced around from job to job for the last thirty years. Some have been for days, weeks, months and some, many years. Ever since I was ten years old, I have worked. I started mowing lawns, raking leaves and shoveling snow. Since then, I have been an actor on TV, dressed as Batman at your kid's birthday party, sold you drinks in a bar, served you food and maybe even performed your wedding. I have sold you everything from a Mercedes, a Christmas tree, a water softener, a talking VCR remote, an 800-toll free #, a phone system for your business, handyman services, Real Estate property to a solar system. And those are only some of the ones I remember! There are many reasons why I chose to get on and ride that career roller coaster, some of which were my choice, because I love a new challenge but, with most, I was just trying to survive. There were many times in my life I was "aware" that something needed to change and I saw all the "obstacles" but what I didn't always have was the best "strategy" or the "execution" to attain my "desired result".

Honestly, I don't have any regrets. I am who I am today because of the choices I have made. But sometimes I wonder, if I had been introduced and coached on how to use this "30

Minute Change" process years ago, where would I be now and how much of the stress, heartache and disappointments could have been avoided. Not to mention all the people I have (pro bono) mentored and coached over the last twenty-five years. But then again, how could I have been trained in a process that had not yet been developed.

Four years ago, an "awareness" came over me. I started immersing myself into researching the brain and why we do what we do. I had reached a new level of frustration with the fact that people around me were not able to make the changes they wanted and needed to make. They had every intention of making the change but could never see it through. I guess this is what keeps psychologists in business. So I set out to specifically understand the conscious and subconscious mind and how they play such a critical role in determining what we do, how we act and what we believe to be true. I have studied the advancement from old Newtonian Physics to the new clarity of Quantum Physics. The "Biology of Belief" by Bruce Lipton was the spark that fueled a lot of this new discovery. I have been trained in New Energy Psychology and have learned how to re-program the subconscious mind (thanks to Rob Williams - Psych-K® and Brain Gym®). The subconscious, by the way, controls 95% of our thoughts every day! I now know that the thoughts we allow in our mind and body can actually cause dire sickness or create miraculous healing. Thankfully, I have learned that we are not controlled by our genes! Rather, the new science known as Epigenetics proves that environmental signals control our genes and that the beliefs and perceptions we allow to enter our lives, individually and collectively, determine our physical biology and ultimately our reality. I have researched the effects of slow mindful breathing and how it can change our physiology and brain waves, as well as having experienced the value of "Whole-Brain" learning and the power it has over our subconscious mind. Finally, I have seen the power of asking deep, thought provoking questions and humbly asking others for help; both of which give us great insight into our Awareness and assist in aligning our universal energy.

Of all that I've studied and learned, one of my favorite teachers throughout my life has been Jesus Christ. He was very in tune with the power of thought and how you can get anything in your life by simply asking for it (with the right motives, of course). Jesus was more amazed by the non-religious people who had simple faith than he ever was by the religious leaders who had tons of knowledge. Let me show you a great example of that. Here we have a story of a women who goes to Jesus to ask for help for her ailing daughter and gets shut down... bigtime.

A Canaanite woman from that vicinity came to him, crying out, "Lord, Son of David, have mercy on me! My daughter is demon-possessed and suffering terribly." Jesus did not answer a word. So, his disciples came to him and urged him, "Send her away, for she keeps crying out after us." Jesus finally answered her, "I was sent only to the lost sheep of Israel." The woman came and knelt before him. "Lord, help me!" she said. He replied, "It is not right to take the children's

5

bread and toss it to the dogs." "Yes it is, Lord," she said. "Even the dogs eat the crumbs that fall from their master's table." Then Jesus said to her, "Woman, you have great faith! Your request is granted." And her daughter was healed at that moment. Matthew 15:22-28 NIV .

The woman knew exactly what she wanted. She had heard about this prophet who was going around healing people. She loved her daughter and was willing to do anything for her. And to her, anything meant even approaching a Jew when she was a Gentile and that was not kosher; hence the disciples telling Jesus to send her away. Then he basically said, "No, I can't help you" twice. She could have walked away after the first rejection, especially after the second, but she did not give up, her daughter's life depended on it. So, she kept asking. Jesus was not annoyed but amazed by her faith!

Faith is a state of mind that is created by our beliefs in the subconscious mind. Simply put, your true thoughts and beliefs will become your faith. This faith will then strengthen your actions which will ultimately create your reality.

One thing I ask as you read this book is for you to be filled with compassion and an understanding of why you are the way you are but, at the same time, feel so empowered that you restore your faith in your ability to make changes in your life instantly. By your New Belief, you will not let what has happened in the past affect your ability to make changes in your future any longer. What you focus on now will determine how you feel, and the questions you ask yourself will control your focus. You just need to make sure you know how to ask the right questions every time to facilitate the desired change. And for those of you who are extremely self-aware and have made incredible changes throughout your life to better yourself and your surroundings, I hope this book will open up a higher level of consciousness through these new skills that will help you define and clarify any new desired change.

Lastly, for those of you who, somewhere along the road of life, decided to pull over and just stay parked; who are not emotionally happy with that choice but have lost the road map and the will to move forward; who, for some reason, have your eyes locked in the rear-view mirror and cannot see past the mistakes being replayed over and over and over again; who no longer believe that your dreams and desires are within reach, so why try...this book will be a new, easy to follow map, that will help get you back on the road for good. I promise!

What is the "30 Minute Change"?

Let me start off by telling you what it is not. It is not a 30-minute routine or program you have to do every day or week. It is not a 30-minute shortcut to lose weight, make money, find love, quit bad habits, start new ones, get in shape or change your career.

The "30 Minute Change" is a One Time detailed step by step process, which engages your current thoughts on a specific subject and then, through a visual, auditory, kinesthetic & Whole-Brain exercise, helps you set a "New Belief Statement"

7

in motion at the subconscious level based on my new formula for change: AOSED.

Awareness + Obstacle + Strategy + Execution = Desired Result.

Let me explain in more detail:

Real and lasting change only happens after personal Awareness begins. Awareness provides a transparent view of the Obstacles. Once you can define the Obstacles, you are able to formulate a Strategy. When you have a clear, detailed Strategy, you are then able to develop your Execution plan. Execution of that plan leads to your Desired Result, also known as your New Belief!

Definitions: Dictionary.com = **D** and Mine = **M**
Awareness:

D - The state or condition of being aware. Having knowledge. Being conscious of.

M - Helps you see where you are at presently. Helps you become aware of things you never knew. Redirects you in the areas of your life where you may be off course and opens the door to your options.

Obstacles:

D – Something that impedes progress or achievement.

M - Self-created road blocks, keeping you from your Desired Result. Misguided thoughts, emotions or feelings you have allowed to stand in the way of achieving your goal.

Strategy:

D - A careful plan or method. The art of devising or employing plans.

M - A detailed Obstacle bulldozer which engages your thoughts, visions, auditory processing and feelings to successfully devise an attainable plan toward the "New Belief"

Execution:

D - The act or process of executing.

M - The immediate steps taken to bring action to your detailed Strategy. The successful forward motion based on your "New Belief" about the Desired Change.

Desired Result:

M - Living out the "New Belief."

How and why this process works!

Imagine being stuck in a dense forest. You know there has to be a way out but, as you are standing there, in the middle, surrounded by hundreds if not thousands of trees and large rocks, the path you should take is just not that clear. Now you could get an emotional feeling and start running in that direction or you could have a thought about which way to go and want to follow that hunch or you could just stand there and listen for any sounds of civilization and, if you think you hear any, head off in that direction or you could look through the trees and try to spot any faint light way off in the distance that could be your guide. Yes! Those are all separate options available at the moment and could, with luck, get you to where you want to go. But what if you could focus your thoughts, your feelings, your audio and visual processors all together at once to help you find your way out. Would that not be more effective and increase your chances of reaching freedom? Yes it would, and that is what I am going to teach you to do with any change you wish to make.

Step One: Awareness
How it works

First, you must take personal responsibility for the situation you want changed. "I want out of the forest!" That is perfect Awareness. From there, everything begins. Without that Awareness, nothing begins. This may sound extremely basic to you but you would be surprised at how many people are "lost in the forest" and have no idea. Sometimes we think we need to be the ones to tell them they are lost. How many times has that backfired on us? I have not yet found a more empowering tool to change than self-awareness. It is like standing in a pitch-black room and having the lights turn on. It's a bit overwhelming at first but shortly leads to perfect clarity. (If you take nothing else away from this book other than the new insight of Awareness, then that will be a great start for you on your journey.) I think you will find Awareness is a simple process and that you will agree that any desired change must indeed start there.

Why it works.

Rather than just having an emotional thought or feeling of, "I think I need to change this in my life" and then moving on to your next thought, Awareness becomes the foundational start to any true and lasting change. When something bothers you enough, you will come to the point when you stop blaming others, stop making excuses, stop trying to justify failed short cuts and accept your personal responsibility to do something about it. When you get to that point, and only then, can the change process begin.

Step Two: Obstacle
How it works

Once you become Aware of the desired or needed change the next step is to take the time to define, evaluate and question the Obstacles. What is keeping you from making this change? This is where many people are misguided. They know there are obstacles in their way and they want to move them or go around them (which is great!) but what happens is, they remove or go around the wrong obstacles. Example: Let's say you want to lose weight. You believe the obstacles are: You don't exercise, eat out too much, don't take vitamins and don't get enough sleep.

But what if you viewed the obstacle like this: You became aware that "I need to lose weight."

What does that mean to you? "I can no longer eat whatever I want, I must be disciplined and conscious of what I buy and order, I must take some decisive action now. I need to change some of the bad eating habits I have, like eating after seven pm."

Why do you want to lose weight? "Because I don't fit in any of my clothes anymore, I feel tired all the time, I have no energy after ten am and I feel stressed a lot."

Why have you gained so much weight? (This is a very deep but essential question to ask yourself here, and your answers may be very personal and lead back to past relationships, hurts or unresolved conflicts.)

If you want to make a real change, you must take the time to question and address the real Obstacles.

Why it works

Getting to know someone on a deeper level involves asking deep questions. Understanding how to improve at your job means asking others questions. In order for the doctor to figure out what ails you, he must ask you questions. Learning is exponentially increased by the amount of questions we ask. Defining what you think the Obstacles are in the wanted change is just the start but by asking the 'who', 'what', 'when', 'where' and 'why' questions to each of those Obstacles, this is the fuel needed to ignite Step Three.

Step Three: Strategy
How it works

As complicated as our brains can seem, they only work in three different stages: The thinking, the doing and the being. I heard Dr. Joe Dispenza talking about this on a Ted Talks and it rang true to everything I have been talking about in the Strategy stage. You will spend the majority of your time in the 'thinking' stage so that the transition to the 'doing' and 'being' will be quite simple. You will be asked to clearly define and engage your mind and body physically, emotionally and mentally in the Strategy. This is what helps to unlock your creative mind to help you think of ways to overcome the defined Obstacles by creating new connections in your brains. Example: Let's first look at your old subconscious way of doing this:

Awareness: "I am in an unhealthy relationship and want out."

Obstacle: "I have been with this person a long time, they will be mad if I leave. I will be alone, what if I am not able to find anyone better?"

Strategy: "Tell him/her we need to take a break."

New, engaged way of making this change.

Awareness: "I am in an unhealthy relationship. I deserve better. I know I am to blame for a big part of why things are the way they are, but I am ready to work on myself."

Obstacle: "I am afraid to be on my own. I am a conflict avoider. I know I need to deal with my junk first before I can be in a healthy, balanced and giving relationship."

Strategy: "Let him/her know that we need to take a long break. That I am not ok with where this relationship is at. That I need the time to work on myself at this time of my life and am seeing things in my character I want and need to change."

* Then you ask yourself "What is the new belief I will have about myself after I do this?" Meaning, once you make the change to end this unhealthy relationship and start to deal with your own junk, what will that New Belief about this change be? Here is an example of your New Belief - "I deserve and welcome only healthy relationships" or, "I love and respect myself

enough to only have healthy relationships." Taking this new Strategy even further, you then physically write down all the pros and cons that will come from making this change to "end this unhealthy relationship". Then, to help program this change, i.e. New Belief, even further into your subconscious belief system, you will now add to this Strategy what this New Belief will actually, look, sound and feel like. Why? Because our subconscious mind only records things it experiences through the five senses. This is where you will physically write down and then begin to experience emotional and mental connection to this New Belief at the subconscious level. This is a technique I learned when I was an actor in College and was learning to memorize lines. I found that when I physically wrote out the lines, visualized them as I was writing and said them out loud to hear them as I was writing, that I was able to memorize three times faster. A simply physiological technique of engaging the key senses. All of these Strategies will be further validated as you delve into the next chapters.

Why it works

By engaging your senses, you will then create new connections and beliefs in your brain. Wikipedia describes "Senses" as: A system that consists of a group of sensory cell types that respond to a specific physical phenomenon, and that corresponds to a particular group of regions within the brain where the signals are received and interpreted.

Have you ever noticed when you are really focused, how

that makes you feel? And when you feel differently, don't you behave differently? This exercise helps you not only focus on what you need to do but why you need to do it, how you need to do it, when you need to do it and how will it look, sound and feel when you do. By doing this, you will be creating sense memories in the hippocampus region of the brain. I know from all the people I have coached through this AOSED change process, not one has ever taken the time to go through their Strategy like this before, ever! It's all about the amount of whole mind and body energy you put into it that helps lock into your subconscious mind the Desired Change. In other words, knowing what to do is just not enough. But if you can also add the experience of what it looks, sounds and feels like to have this New Belief, you will actually train your brain to create new circuitry, new firing patterns, new sequences and ultimately a new program.

Step Four: Execution
How it works

Now that you have taken the time to define and participate in your Strategy, the next step is to Execute. Again, this must be clearly defined and built off of your Strategy. If you were to look back over previous failures (though I hate that word because there is no real failure if you learned from it), you will see that on many occasions it was because of the lack of Execution. Some will say it was lack of effort but I say that if the effort was not spent on the Strategy then the effort towards Execution will fall short as well. The Execution is taking the

Strategy and adding detailed action and a specific timeline to each defined Strategy. Based on the example above, the Strategy is: "Let him/her know that we need to take a break. That I am not ok with where this relationship is at. That I need the time to work on myself at this time in my life and am seeing things in my character I want and need to change."

The Execution would look like this:

- Call him/her and set a time to be alone and talk where there will be no distractions.
- Think through and write out exactly what I am feeling and want to say.
- Admit my part in all of this and explain I am getting some help to work through some things.
- Do not talk to him/her for at least two weeks.
- Download and read the book Boundaries that my mother has been telling me about.
- Seek advice on where to get some help with my trust issues.

After you have defined your Execution plan, you will then clarify your New Belief about this change you are making and how it will make you feel about and believe about yourself. It may be slightly different from the New Belief statement you first made in Step Three. The new statement is: "I love and respect myself enough to only have healthy relationships."

Why it works

By this step in the process, once learned, you are about

twenty-five minutes into the desired change. You are Aware of what needs to change, you are crystal clear on the Obstacles and you are all in on the Strategy. So, the Execution is just taking what you have laid out before you and putting defined actions and timelines to it. There is no confusion at this point, you are not relying on emotions or random thoughts to help you implement here, you are just applying actions to your Strategies.

Step Five: Desired Result = New Belief
How it works.

Your thoughts are at the conscious level, which is your creative mind. Your beliefs are at the subconscious level, your habitual mind, that runs programs, most of which are self-sabotaging or limited by what you saw, heard or felt as a child. Here is where you'll reprogram your subconscious mind to accept your New Belief about the Desired Change. This is done with Whole-Brain Programming.

I use energy work called the Whole-Brain Posture. This is where you sit comfortably in a chair crossing your feet at the ankles, right over left and then hold your arms out in front of you, palms facing outwards, cross them at the wrist, left over right with the thumbs facing down, now your palms will be facing each other and you simply clasp your palms together and drop them in your lap and relax. Then you place the tip of your tongue behind your upper front teeth. The governing and central meridians meet at the part behind the upper front teeth, but there is a little gap. The tongue helps close that gap.

The action of having your limbs crossed over integrates the left and right hemispheres of the brain. Your left side analyzes using logic and reason. Your right side synthesizes using emotion and intuition. Normally each hemisphere operates interdependently, although the brain's natural function is to use both hemispheres simultaneously, often stresses or emotionally charged experiences can be stored in only one hemisphere. Subsequently therefore the brain may over identify with only the side of the brain that had that similar experience and now we want to go in there and tell it to believe something it doesn't know to be true? Just because you consciously believe, want and need to make this change doesn't mean your subconscious will. The programs may be at odds with one another: the new thought may be in conflict with the thought of what has been ingrained at an earlier stage of life. That is why, when we cross over the hemispheres, we can help unlock the subconscious brain to accept the New Belief. (Note. This will not happen without the details and experiences of the first four steps above, all of which prime the subconscious to accept the New Belief.)

Then, while you're in this relaxed position, I will have you close your eyes and begin to repeat your New Belief (Example: "I love and respect myself enough to only have healthy relationships.") over and over silently in your mind until you experience a mental, emotional or physical change in your mind and body about your New Belief. After a few minutes you will feel a change in your thoughts, feelings or emotions. Then you open your eyes, uncross your body and Lock in the New Belief by holding your hands in front of you in a prayer position for a few seconds. That's it! The New Belief has been programmed into your subconscious. You just need to go and live out your New Belief by Executing your Strategy. Then, whenever your conscious mind repeats the old negative patterns about that belief, you just remind it of your newly created and subconsciously programmed New Belief statement.

Why it works.

This is not an affirmation which is a conscious thought, rather this is a New Belief that will be programmed and accepted into your subconscious mind. Big difference! We have all tried affirmations, telling ourselves in the mirror every morning when we wake up, "I am happy and successful", "Money comes to me", "I am secure and confident", "I am worthy of a better job", "I am thin and beautiful" etc... Those are great conscious thoughts, but the problem is that the programs that run your mind, thoughts and actions do not believe or accept those conscious thoughts. The conscious mind is creative, lives in the moment and dreams of the future. It controls about 5% of your brain. The subconscious, which operates 95% of the brain, runs programs like your bodily functions and nervous system, it controls your biology, your habits, your past learned emotions, your true beliefs about things and your past learned patterns and thoughts. So you can stand in front of the mirror all day long and tell yourself you are thin and beautiful but if your subconscious believes and is programmed from your childhood that you are "not as pretty as your sister" or you will "never live up to your parents expectations", then it doesn't matter what you say. I am not saying all affirmations are a waste of time. It has been proven that affirmation will work if you do it enough times for extended periods of time, maybe years in some cases. You are welcome to take years to do that if you wish. But what I am talking about with this change process is creating New Beliefs at the subconscious level. Recording new thoughts into the programs that run your brain. Using proven techniques that will help you experience this amazing change today.

Just getting back to the beginning of who we were made to be:

There is an ancient proverb that says, "You cannot bring out of a person what is not already instilled within them." That being said, your ability to change is naturally ingrained into who you are at the core. Don't let the things that have happened in your past take away the power of your future. As you will discover in this book, most changes in your life are instantaneous and have always been that way. From the day you were born, you were actually hard wired with the AOSED formula already installed in your brain. You didn't have to think very hard about what you wanted back then in order to get it. Something inside you just kicked in and, before you knew what was happening, you were receiving your desired results.

For Example:

Let's look at a newborn, helpless little baby (so we think) and how they obtain food.

What's the Awareness? They are hungry.

The Obstacle? They have no food and can't feed themselves.

The Strategy? Get the attention of someone who will feed them.

The Execution? They cry.

The Desired Result? Someone gives them food.

Again...we are preprogrammed to overcome Obstacles!

Now let's look at a toddler (two-three years old) who has just woken up in the playpen after his nap.

- **Awareness:** He wants out.
- **Obstacle:** He can't get out himself.
- **Strategy:** Get picked up or let out!
- **Execution:** Cry, scream or yell.
- **Desired Result:** He gets picked up.

Again...we are preprogrammed to overcome obstacles!

This process is not only used to get what we want but, as we age, we begin to use this process for safety, protection or even deception.

Let's take the third-grade girl who's afraid to give the wrong answer in class.

- **Awareness:** She does not want to look stupid in front of her classmates.
- **Obstacle:** Her teacher knows she is smart and wants to call on her.
- **Strategy:** To not get called on.
- **Execution:** She does not raise her hand or make eye contact with her teacher.
- **Desired Result:** The teacher calls on someone else.

Again...we are preprogrammed to overcome the obstacles in our lives.

What about the teenager who wants to stay out past his curfew?

- **Awareness:** He wants to stay out later than he can, like all his friends do.
- **Obstacle:** If he does, he will get grounded next weekend.
- **Strategy:** Convince his parents to let him stay with a friend who is going through a hard time and needs him.
- **Execution:** Come up with a believable story, call his mom and tell it to her.
- **Desired Result:** She decides to let him stay over at his friend's house.

Or the campus student who wants to stay in school.

- **Awareness:** If her grades don't improve, she will get kicked out of school.
- **Obstacle:** Between parties and friends, there is no time to study.
- **Strategy:** Focus on school for the next month to pass all her finals.
- **Execution:** She makes excuses to her friends and forces herself to go to the library every day.
- **Desired Result:** She passes the classes and gets to stay in school

There are thousands of other examples I could give here, but you get the point. These are all very natural progressions we go through and have always gone through to get what we wanted...or in some cases what we didn't want. The problem lies sometime between our childhood and now. Somewhere along the road we gave up on this natural "healthy" process of overcoming obstacles: Awareness + Obstacle + Strategy + Execution = Desired Result. Instead, subconsciously, we created our own process for dealing with change. For many of us it now looks like this:

Obstacle + **Avoid**: always going around + **Deny**: pretend it's not there + **Procrastinate**: one day I will make the change + **Excuse**: if only "this" would happen, then I would change + **Complain**: it's just too hard to make changes = **Undesired Result.**

I am not here to be your therapist, I do not believe you need to trudge through your whole past to change your future. I have always believed that: living in the past is depressive and living in the future cause's anxiety (Awareness tip: If you find yourself feeling depressed, you're probably living in the past. If you find yourself struggling with anxiety, then you are trying to live in the future). Personally, I believe God gave us "today" only; to live in, control and have the ability to change this day alone. We cannot change the past and we cannot control the future, *although things we do today, can and will adjust our future.* I also believe that it doesn't have to take days, weeks or months to change negative or destructive beliefs in your life. I know for a fact you can alter the outcome of your future in 30

23

minutes or less by doing the exercises I am about to show you in this book. I use this "30 Minute Change" technique to help coach individuals and organizations in all different areas of need: Personal Growth, Health & Fitness, Relationships, Finances, Marriage, Parenting, Hobbies, Weight, Career advancement, etc...

Whether you initially agree with my next statement or not is up to you, but I believe the more that you let it settle in and then test it, the harder it will be to deny:

"We are all made up of the things we've seen, the things we've heard and the feelings we've had. These then become the foundation of how we now see things, hear things and feel things and, by default, will determine our thoughts about any current situation in our life."

Why change doesn't work for most people.

Studies show that the average person makes the same New Year's resolution eight years in a row. However, most of these year-beginning promises to ourselves are left by the wayside within the first six weeks, leaving some of us to ask, "Why is change so difficult...and does it have to be?" I say NO, and will spend the rest of this book showing you why. However, there is another force fighting to tell you otherwise: multiple industries make their living from the fact that most people believe change is too hard and so these industries in turn rely on that belief for their future revenue stream. Just open a magazine, turn on the TV or spend any time on the internet to prove that point.

Nowadays it seems like everything out there is telling us we need to change. There are thousands if not hundreds of thousands of books, DVD's, videos, classes, TV commercials, workshops, seminars and retreats that will help us change this or that in our lives. So, what that conveys is that the human race is always evolving, people are always looking to improve themselves and constantly trying to live up to their true potential. I know I am, and I am so thrilled to be living in a world where there are many tools available for helping me to do so. The one thing I have noticed though, is that most of those plans are about wanting you to rely on someone or something else to make the change. What's different about the "30 Minute Change" is that it's about empowering <u>your</u> thoughts, i.e. <u>your</u> belief system, back to its originally designed state of being. Once you learn and put into practice the techniques taught to you in this new process, you will be able to make almost any Desired Change in your life in "30 Minutes or Less". You will not necessarily need to join a support group, go to a weeklong seminar, pay to see motivational speakers, read a book a week on the subject, etc.... to make any of these changes. Unless, of course, you choose one of those as your Strategies to facilitate the needed change, which is perfectly fine. More on that later!

Throughout the next few chapters I will break down each change category with examples and specific processes to facilitate the desired change. All that is required from you is to <u>trust</u> the process. Learning is improved by repetitive patterns. That is why there are so many examples in each chapter. Once you understand the meaning behind the patterns you are about to learn, you will then enter a higher consciousness with regard to make lasting changes in your life. You will get out what you put into this change process. A well-known study shows that 70% of what we learn, we learn by doing, 20% by exchanging ideas and only 10% by seeing. If you read this book without implementing the procedures outlined in it, you will limit your experience to some new insights. If on the other hand, once you take the time to learn, process the questions, write down your answers and physically engage in the Whole-Brain exercises, you will be able to experience life changing results as soon as today!!

Chapter 1

Personal Growth

"People always ask me...why does this "30 Minute Change" process work
So well? I tell them, because everything you have ever seen, heard or felt in
Your past, Determines how you see, hear and feel things presently, so if
You can <u>learn</u> how to see, hear and feel things differently today, those New
Beliefs will create for you, a new tomorrow."

It took me a long time to decide which "change" process I wanted to start this book with. Initially I felt like, "Let's start with something fun like 'Defining and Finding your Dream Job' or 'Creating New Hobbies', those are a blast to do!" But then, the more I thought about it and looked at the facts (we will talk about facts versus feelings later in the book), the reality was that even those fun chapters all start with Personal Growth. How can you take a massive step towards going after your Dream Job without changing some of your core beliefs about yourself? How can you decide to jump faithfully into a New Hobby if you don't conquer your fear and build confidence? How can you work on changes in your Relationships without changing you first? How can you work on your Health or Fitness without defining what that means to you personally in your own life? How do you change your Financial situation without first seeing what personally is causing the problem?

Catch my drift? They all lead back to the foundation of our core being. Why we feel like we feel, why we think how we think, why we act like we act, why we see things as we see them. The common phrase being, what we think about, we ultimately bring about. Or, as I like to say, everything you have ever seen, heard or felt in your past, determines how you see, hear and feel things today.

As a child for the first six or seven years of your life, you were just a sponge, soaking up everything you saw, heard and felt. The cognitive part of your brain was not fully developed so your ability to question the things you saw and heard and felt was limited, mostly, to how it made you feel. You were not able to process the why and then recognize the thought patterns that made you feel that way. Yes, you knew ice cream was amazing and the feeling you experienced when you ate it was ecstasy, but when you parents, teacher, coach, sibling, etc... told you that you were bad, lazy, dumb, or mean. You were not able to process that they may just be having a bad day and didn't really mean it or that is something someone told them when they were little so they thought it was OK to tell you. You just believed what you were told. You brain was just recording everything. That is why most of the current problems in your life now stem from your earlier programed subconscious thoughts and beliefs. This is why it is so important to create and record new empowering beliefs over the old ones and this is done with the new "30 Minute Change" AOSED process.

Some of the other change processes described in the next chapters will be done on a weekly, monthly, yearly or possibly a one-time change cycle. Personal growth, however, is something you will be working on changing for the rest of your life, so that is why I am going to start here. After helping you become aware of how simple this AOSED change process is and by providing you with some engaging tools, you will be able to clearly define and succeed with your Desired Change.

It is simple and will work every time...if you only believe. The good news is, no one controls your beliefs, except you. Nothing and no one can keep you from achieving your Desired Belief Change...except you. If just saying that is not enough to convince you, then I will help, by teaching you to "overcome you"!

Let's Begin:

Again, the dictionary defines awareness as: the state or condition of being aware; having knowledge; being conscious of.

What a perfect and essential place to start the Desired Change process, although, in this book, we are going to focus on taking it a step further: Self-awareness. Face it, it's very easy to be aware of all the things everyone else needs to change. We don't need any help learning how to do that. We can see all the problems with the people and the world around us and in most cases the reason why they are that way. Believe me, we were all born with the gift of criticalness, which we justify as "insight". Anytime we give our power away to something or someone outside ourselves, we automatically disconnect from the control of our inner world, where true change happens, and empower the outer world, over which we have absolutely no control (no matter how much we think we may). I believe what we've lost along our "journey of life" is our deep need for self-awareness and the empowering guidance that comes with it. When we choose to listen to and accept our state of awareness, we will deepen the levels of consciousness where inner guidance and clarity abound.

One of the things that hinders us most from personal growth is our "falsely trusted" ability to judge others against ourselves. For many of us this was subconsciously programed in from birth, then carried on throughout our schooling and into our current phase of life as well:

- Why aren't you as smart as your sister?
- David doesn't do that!
- When I was a kid, my mother never let me get away with that.
- D minus....no one in this family has ever even got a D.
- See the way she wears her hair, why don't you do yours like that?
- You're just like your father!
- Why don't you go outside and play sports with the neighborhood boys, what's wrong with you?
- If you don't go to college you will be doing manual labor for the rest of your life.
- Your father really hoped you were going to be a boy.
- Your mother has never been the same since you were born.

- If I never had you kids, I would have been _____!

Or maybe at work you have heard:

- This is Jack, our best salesman, try to be like him.

- Samar over there, she works late every night... and she has kids.

- If you don't do it exactly like this, you will need to find a new job.

- If only you had gone to that college, then you would be promoted.

- The guy you are replacing was very detailed and turned his projects in days before deadline, but no pressure!

- Why would you want to stay home with your baby, you know you'll never get a shot at that promotion if you do.

- It's not that you're lying, you're just stretching the truth a bit.

- If it was me, I would do it this way.

- You weren't hired for your ability to think, we just need you to follow the process.

And we wonder why it's hard to make personal growth changes in our lives. Holy Cow!!! Do you see any of these ringing true in your life? Can you hear these being repeated in your head? Did you feel a little sick inside when you read those? I know I did, even writing them.

I know we all have skeletons buried in the closet and I am not saying we need to open the door wide and let them all out. But, in order to make personal changes, we have to become aware of what is causing the "standstill" on this much needed change. So, what I am suggesting here is, you just crack open the closet, use the small light on your cell phone and look for the one or two things that will help you address the Obstacles that stand in your way of creating a New Belief for a particular needed change.

Alright, now it's time to walk you through the AOSED Change process and show you how empowering this is to assist you with the Desired Change. I am going to start off with a "very simple" change and then we will work our way into the deep end. Welcome to the "30 Minute **Change**" process: Below are some examples for Personal Growth.

1. Needed Change: I Watch Too Much TV

You have probably been thinking about this for a while but now you are ready to actually do **something** about it.

PERSONAL GROWTH CHANGE
PROCESS FORM

THE AWARENESS: (MUST BE PERSONAL AND DETAILED.)

I don't have much of a life. I work then I come home and turn on the TV. There is nothing on Netflix I haven't seen. That is very scary!

THE OBSTACLE: (MUST BE CLEARLY DETAILED AND DEFINED.)

I am tired after work and it's easy to veg on the couch. Once I get into a show I have to watch them all. It makes it too easy without the commercials. I forgot what I used to do before all this. I am not sure what I would do with all that extra time.

THE STRATEGY: (MUST BE THOUGHT OUT, DETAILED AND COMMITTED TO.)

Limit the amount I watch. Find other things to do. Don't go home after work.

WHAT IS THE NEW BELIEF YOU WANT TO HAVE?

(THIS IS A ROUGH DRAFT THOUGHT HERE. YOU WILL CLARIFY LATER IN THE PROCESS.)

I don't need to live my life through the characters on TV. I can have my life back or create a new one.

Pros of This Choice	Cons of This Choice
Spend time with friends	*Will miss my shows*
Get some hobbies	*Forced to be social*
Lose weight	*Will need to do something*
Have a social life	
Get into a relationship	
Finish my projects	
Read a book	
Start a business	
Help out my neighbors	
Go hiking	
Write some letters	
Call some old friends	
Take a cooking class	
Join the Gym	

(Take your time and write down as many Pros and Cons as you can think of! This helps solidify why this New Belief is valuable to you.)

WHAT THAT NEW STRATEGY LOOKS, SOUNDS AND FEELS LIKE.

Take a moment and close your eyes. Picture yourself already living out this New Belief.
Then describe in detail what you see, hear and feel.

Visual (I see...)

- *I see myself coming home, changing into my workout clothes and going to the gym.*
- *I see myself sitting at a coffee shop reading a book and meeting new people.*

33

- *I see myself sitting on a plane with my friends going on vacation to Hawaii.*

Auditory (I hear...)

- *I hear the sound of the birds and the wind as I walk along the hiking trail.*
- *I hear the new neighbor I met knocking on my door to hang out.*
- *I hear my mom thanking me for calling her so often and asking her about her.*

Kinesthetic (I feel...)

- *I feel refreshed. I feel more energetic. I feel in tune with the real world around me.*

THE EXECUTION: (MUST BE TIED TO YOUR STRATEGY AND PUT INTO MOTION IMMEDIATELY)

I will limit myself to two Hours of TV and internet a day. I will go to the gym after work to get signed up. I will say hello to my neighbors and try to start a conversation getting to know them. I will go online to sign up for a cooking class during my break at work today. I will find at least one new hobby.

THE DESIRED RESULT: (YOUR NEW PERSONAL BELIEF STATEMENT)

I am in control of my life and can do new and exciting things.

WHOLE-BRAIN PROGRAMING: (This adds the New Belief to your subconscious. Before starting this final exercise, read though your whole change process form one more time.)

Get into a Whole-Brain Posture (sitting on a chair, legs and arms crossed).
Close your eyes and think about your new desired result belief statement.

"I am in control of my life and can do new and exciting things."

Concentrate on experiencing a mental, emotional or physical change in your mind and body about your New Belief statement as you repeat it over and over again silently.

After a few minutes you will feel a change in your thoughts, feelings or emotions.

Then open your eyes, uncross your body and lock in the New Belief.

See appendix A in the back of this book for the detailed process of how to do the "Whole-Brain Programing" exercise.

Note: The Whole-Brain Posture is inspired by a Brain Gym® activity called Hook-ups. Brain Gym is a registered trademark of the Educational Kinesiology Foundation in Santa Barbara CA, USA.

2. Needed change: Negativity

Let's say you became aware that you are a very negative person. Again, this will not work if other people think you are negative, it will only work if you become aware that you believe you're negative. Now let's personalize this even further. First off, let me say you are not a negative person, for is there really such a thing? But rather you choose to see most things in a negative way, you tend to speak and hear most things in a negative fashion and you feel negative towards most things, most of the time. Breaking it down and clearly defining the Desired Change is very important. You cannot change you as a person because that is too broad but now that you have broken it down, you can change the way you see things, control the way you speak, adjust how you hear things and learn to feel differently about being negative. It's learning to ask yourself the right questions.

PERSONAL GROWTH CHANGE
PROCESS FORM

THE AWARENESS: (MUST BE PERSONAL AND DETAILED)

I am really negative! I choose to focus on the negative things going on around me. People have been telling me this for a while, but I always seem to have an excuse. My negative thinking keeps me from deep relationships. The opposite of negative is positive.

THE OBSTACLE: (MUST BE CLEARLY DETAILED AND DEFINED)

I have a hard time trusting people because I have been hurt in the past. I do this to protect myself from having unfulfilled expectations. I mostly hang around other negative people. I find it easier to complain than do something about it.

THE STRATEGY: (MUST BE THOUGHT OUT, DETAILED AND COMMITTED TO)

I will keep my negative thoughts to myself. I will look deeper at the cause of each negative thought and try to separate it from the others. I will spend less time being around negative people. I will say at least one positive thing to each person I have a conversation with. I will read a book about being positive to make sure I keep my focus.

WHAT IS THE NEW BELIEF YOU WANT TO HAVE?
(THIS IS A ROUGH DRAFT THOUGHT HERE. YOU WILL CLARIFY LATER IN THE PROCESS.)

That I can be a positive person. I look on the bright side of things. I stop and think before I complain about anything.

Pros of This Choice:	*Cons of This Choice:*
Find more peace	*Will have to work hard at this*
Enjoy life more often	*Can't make excuses anymore*
Not be so angry	*Will need to get out of myself*
See things a different way	*May lose some of my friends*
Learn to forgive	
Not feel so guilty	
Be happy	
Probably get promoted	
Help others who are negative	
Look for the good	
Improve my relationships	

(Take your time and write down as many Pros and Cons as you

can think of! This helps solidify why this New Belief is valuable to you.)

WHAT THAT NEW STRATEGY LOOKS, SOUNDS AND FEELS LIKE.

Take a moment and close your eyes. Picture yourself already living out this New Belief.
Then describe in detail what you see, hear and feel.

Visual (I see...)

I see myself taking a batch of cookies to my (not so nice) neighbor James

I see myself walk in the house and greet my family smiling without being critical that things are not how I wish them.

I see myself complimenting one person about one good thing every day.

Auditory (I hear...)

I hear my friend Maria from the office walking over and tell me how much I have changed and how positive I am.

I hear my boyfriend complimenting me how nice I was to that store clerk.

I hear my son say "I forgive you mom" after I apologize for being so down on him all the time.

Kinesthetic (I feel...)

I feel encouraging. I feel refreshed and alive. I feel the energy from being around like minded positive people.

THE EXECUTION: (MUST BE TIED TO YOUR STRATEGY AND PUT INTO MOTION IMMEDIATELY)

Today I will compliment Jane at work, Keith the UPS guy and call and say nice things to my mom. I will stop at the bookstore on the way home and find a book on staying positive. When I feel like complaining, I will take a deep breath and think about the day my son was born -the best memory I have.

THE DESIRED RESULT: (YOUR NEW PERSONAL BELIEF STATEMENT)

I am a joyful happy person who looks for the good in all things.

WHOLE-BRAIN PROGRAMING: (This adds the New Belief to your subconscious. Before starting this final exercise, read though your whole change process form one more time.)

Get into a Whole-Brain Posture (sitting on a chair, legs and arms crossed). Close your eyes and think about your new desired result belief statement.

"I am a joyful happy person who looks for the good in all things."

Concentrate on experiencing a mental, emotional or physical change in your mind and body about your New Belief statement as you repeat it over and over again silently.
After a few minutes you will feel a change in your thoughts, feelings or emotions.
Then open your eyes, uncross your body and lock in the New Belief.

3. Needed change: Procrastination

So, you finally became aware that you tend to procrastinate and it has led you to the point where you have surrendered to actually doing something about it.

PERSONAL GROWTH CHANGE PROCESS FORM

THE AWARENESS: (MUST BE PERSONAL AND DETAILED)

If I had a $100 for every time I said I would do something and didn't, I would be retired. My ability to procrastinate is hurting my wife and kids. They see me as a big talker. This is the reason I am stuck where I am at work. Now that I think about it, a lot of my anger stems from this area of my life. I need to change this once and for all!

THE OBSTACLE: (MUST BE CLEARLY DETAILED AND DEFINED)

I am afraid to fail. Deep down I am lazy and set in my ways. I lack self-discipline, I don't know where to start, I have so many unfinished projects.

THE STRATEGY: (MUST BE THOUGHT OUT, DETAILED AND COMMITTED TO)

I will think before I speak. I will not start a new project until I finish the previous one. I will seek advice from friends and family on how I can improve this part of my life. I will watch a few YouTube videos on being self-disciplined.

WHAT IS THE NEW BELIEF YOU WANT TO HAVE?
(THIS IS A ROUGH DRAFT THOUGHT HERE. YOU WILL CLARIFY LATER IN THE PROCESS.)

I will do what I say or I won't even say it. I do things for others and complete each project I start.

Pros of This Choice	*Cons of This Choice*
I feel good about myself	*Not as much free time*
My wife is happy	*No more excuses*
I accomplish a lot	*Can't be lazy*
I will get the job I want	
My garage is clean	
I will find all my old stuff	
My kids want to spend time with me	
The value of my home will increase	
I sleep peacefully	
I am doing what I love to do	
I am in better health	
My dream of going to Alaska to fish will come true	

(Take your time and write down as many Pros and Cons as you can think of! This helps solidify why this New Belief is valuable to you.)

WHAT THAT NEW STRATEGY LOOKS, SOUNDS AND FEELS LIKE.

Take a moment and close your eyes. Picture yourself already

living out this New Belief.
Then describe in detail what you see, hear and feel.

Visual (I see...)

- *I see myself walking into the garage and everything is where it belongs*
- *I see my wife and kids waiting outside to go to the park together after work*
- *I see myself sitting watching the game with a beer in my hand under the new patio cover I completed.*

Auditory (I hear...)

- *I hear my wife telling me how proud she is of my spending so much time with the kids*
- *I hear my boss telling me I am getting a raise*
- *I hear my daughter asking me if she can sit on my lap and read her a story.*

Kinesthetic (I feel...)

- *I feel unstoppable. I feel united with my family again. I feel no more guilt about not doing what I said I would.*

THE EXECUTION: (MUST BE TIED TO YOUR STRATEGY AND PUT INTO MOTION IMMEDIATELY)

I will ask my wife tonight what is the most important thing I can do for her around the house. I will take the family to the park after work tomorrow for a picnic. I will stop and get their favorite drinks and snacks. I will set aside the whole day Saturday to clean the garage and attic. I will ask my wife if I can start putting $100 a month away for my Alaska fishing trip.

THE DESIRED RESULT: (YOUR NEW PERSONAL BELIEF STATEMENT)

I am successfully united with my family and myself, and do what I say I will do.

WHOLE-BRAIN PROGRAMING: (This adds the New Belief to your subconscious. Before starting this final exercise, read though your whole change process form one more time.)

Get into a Whole-Brain Posture (sitting on a chair, legs and arms crossed).
Close your eyes and think about your new desired result belief statement.

"I am successfully united with my family and myself, and do what I say I will do"

Concentrate on experiencing a mental, emotional or physical change in your mind and body about your New Belief statement as you repeat it over and over again silently.
After a few minutes you will feel a change in your thoughts, feelings or emotions.
Then open your eyes, uncross your body and lock in the New Belief.

4. Needed change: I Don't Deserve Good Things.

I have saved the easiest change for last. (Lol) Most people believe this is one of the hardest things to change and, if that belief is true for them, the change will never happen. On the other hand, if you believe the change can be easily made, then that belief will be true for you. The programs for this limiting belief run deep and you may have been programmed along the way with: "Man, you had a screwed-up childhood, no wonder you're the way you are." or, "I see now why you always feel so bad about yourself." or, "It's ok to feel that way, you had a rough childhood".

Whether it was these or other affirmations just like them, at some point you chose to accept that programming into your subconscious which means your past is now defining your future. Please don't get me wrong here, I am in no way saying you did this as a self-sacrifice or that it was a self-inflicted choice. You did it as a coping mechanism and a survival tool.

You most likely were not aware it even happened but you have been living with its outcome for as long as you can remember. I know, because I have lived it, to some degree, myself.

My parents changed my Parochial school when I was in 4th grade so I went from a school where everyone knew me and I was the cool kid, to a new school where I knew nobody and was not cool.

The first day at the new school, someone went and told the popular kid in my grade that "there's this new kid in school who looks just like you!" Well that popular kid, let's just call him Rick, since I can't remember his real name, decided at that moment that he didn't like me and went and got one of the foreign exchange students at the school to walk over and punch me square in the face. So that was the first day of my new school. Over the next few weeks, Rick was able to orchestrate a coup against me and started the "Sweeney Hate Club". He actually had all the kids sign up on a sheet. There were only two boys that did not sign the sheet. So, let's just say that was a brutal school year. I had girls that were friends of Rick's walk up and kick me in the privates. I had to fight three or four times a month. I got kicked out of two of the fourth-grade classes and would have been kicked out of school but one teacher took pity on me. When we went to church events, I spent the whole time hiding from the gang of kids that wanted to kick my butt. I told no one, my parents and my teachers just thought I was a trouble maker. Praise God I got out of that school after one year and was able to go the local neighborhood school with my friends.

I did not realize the massive effect that this had on me for the rest of my life until my late thirties. What happened subconsciously was, I became so consumed with what people thought of me that there was no way I could let anybody "not like me". I became a chameleon. Whatever I needed to do to fit in and be accepted I did: I was a habitual liar, I used people to get what I wanted, I became completely self-consumed. It's probably why becoming an actor was such an easy and satisfying transition in college. So, from the time I was in 5th grade until my late thirties, I subconsciously lived this way. Not that I am 100% cured, but I became aware and was able to make drastic changes. Not to mention I had an amazing spiritual experience at twenty-five that helped me work through a lot of these issues even though I was not yet able to pinpoint the cause, like I was able to do with this "Change Process". Let me be clear, I am not saying my life trap was as drastic as yours but, in my mind, what I had seen, heard, felt and from what I subconsciously believed, it was.

Now back to overcoming the lie of: **I Don't Deserve Good Things.**

What I have learned over the years is that this is a big issue for those with challenging childhoods. I have also learned that if you are willing to be totally honest and vulnerable with yourself through this process and willing to do the work, you will be able to initiate the change of this limiting belief.

PERSONAL GROWTH CHANGE PROCESS FORM

THE AWARENESS: (MUST BE PERSONAL AND DETAILED)

I do deserve to have a great life. I am sick of living in the land of crap! I want to live in the moment and be at peace.

THE OBSTACLE: (MUST BE CLEARLY DETAILED AND DEFINED)

I believe I don't deserve good things to happen in my life. I think they are great for everyone else, just not me. Bad things always seem to follow me. I dwell on the past. If good things happen to me they will quickly be taken away.

THE STRATEGY: (MUST BE THOUGHT OUT, DETAILED AND COMMITTED TO)

Spend time each day thinking about things that make me happy. I will find a way to focus on my strengths and do something for someone else. Spend time in prayer and meditation each morning. Create a new belief about myself starting today and repeat it until I believe it. Spoil myself.

WHAT IS THE NEW BELIEF YOU WANT TO HAVE?
(THIS IS A ROUGH DRAFT THOUGHT HERE. YOU WILL CLARIFY LATER IN THE PROCESS.)

I deserve to have a wonderful life, filled with good people and good things

Pros of This Choice	*Cons of This Choice*
I feel good about myself	*I am afraid*
My friends are happy for me	*Can't make excuses*
I am out of my comfort zone	*This will be uncomfortable*
There will be endless possibilities	*My mom may judge me*
I will find a new boyfriend who sees the new me.	
I can forgive myself	
I can forgive my parents	
This will help me stop therapy	
I will sleep peacefully	
I can dream big for the first time	
Everything will be new for me	
No more victim mindset	

(Take your time write and down as many Pros and Cons as you can think of! This helps solidify why this New Belief is valuable to you.)

WHAT THAT NEW STRATEGY LOOKS, SOUNDS AND FEELS LIKE.

44

Take a moment and close your eyes. Picture yourself already living out this New Belief.

Then describe in detail what you see, hear and feel.

Visual (I see...)

- *I see myself sitting on the couch with my friends laughing*
- *I see myself all dressed up at a nice restaurant with my handsome new boyfriend*
- *I see myself looking in the mirror and smiling at the wonderful person I see.*

Auditory (I hear...)

- *I hear my friend Sherri telling me "It's amazing, it's like you're a new person."*
- *I hear the hostess ask me where I got my beautiful stylish shoes*
- *I hear my father tell me how proud he is of me and that he has always loved me.*

Kinesthetic (I feel...)

- *I feel content. I feel like I belong in this world and I serve a great purpose.*

THE EXECUTION: (MUST BE TIED TO YOUR STRATEGY AND PUT INTO MOTION IMMEDIATELY)

I will write myself a letter listing at least twenty-five good qualities I have and send it to myself in the mail. I will set aside $50 a week and then take myself shopping at the end of each month for a new pair of shoes. Get up half an hour early ever morning to read something inspiring, pray and meditate on my strengths. By the end of the week I will have found a volunteer program to spend time with those less fortunate than myself.

THE DESIRED RESULT: (YOUR NEW PERSONAL BELIEF STATEMENT.)

I have an incredible life and love and accept myself just as I am.

WHOLE-BRAIN PROGRAMING: (This adds the New Belief to your subconscious. Before starting this final exercise, read though your whole change process form one more time.)

45

Get into a Whole-Brain Posture (sitting on a chair, legs and arms crossed).
Close your eyes and think about your new desired result belief statement.

"I have an incredible life and love & accept myself just as I am."

Concentrate on experiencing a mental, emotional or physical change in your mind and body about your New Belief statement as you repeat it over and over again silently.
After a few minutes you will feel a change in your thoughts, feelings or emotions.
Then open your eyes, uncross your body and lock in the New Belief.

I am not sure what changes you would like to make as far as your own Personal Growth is concerned; they may be heavy like a few of those examples above or they may be very light like:

- I am a pack rat
- I don't get enough sleep
- I am too messy
- I want to move to a better area
- I want to meet my neighbors
- I want to be a better listener
- I would like some new friends
- I want to be more organized
- I need to add more reading into my routine
- I want to go back to school and get a degree in _____!
- Etc....

Whatever you choose, be sure to break it down from the

start. If you say "I need to be more disciplined." Why? What does that really mean to you, to "be more disciplined"? Is it because someone told you that? Is it because you hear the words of your deceased father over and over again in the back of your mind? Did you read about it how important it is to be disciplined in a book? Or is it because you are starting to see the damage being undisciplined is causing in your life right now? If you can start there, it only gets better!

The changes you will make by taking the time to go through one of these exercises will amaze you. You can take out a piece of paper and do this anytime you want to make a change or if you would like to download a set of "Change Process" forms that are already created for you to just fill in, they are available for download at: **www30MinuteChange.com**

Bonus: If you feel like you need some extra help getting started on any of the change processes in this book, we offer a one on one personal coaching session available for you. It is a focused 90-minute training session done over the phone. Your coach will help walk you through one or two needed changes in detail. The ultimate goal of this session is to train and equip you with the ability to take yourself through any of your needed change processes in 30 minutes or less going forward. This is a great "one time" training option for some and has had tremendous success. For more info:

Visit: www.30MinuteChange.com

*(I would like to state that people suffering from mental illness or on some doctor ordered prescriptions, as well as certain addicts, may not experience the same results.)

Chapter 2

Define and Find Your Dream Job

*"Find out what you truly love to do and then direct all your
Beliefs towards doing it. Just remember that what you believe
Must in some way benefit those around you."*

I believe that you will find this next chapter very insightful and it will help you to dive into new depths of self-awareness with regard to what you should be doing with your life. The Desired Result will be you sailing off into the sunset with your perfect Dream Job, the one that you were meant to get up for every morning. Let me start off by saying that if you love your current employment and believe you are actually working in your "Dream Job", then please skip this chapter and focus your energy on another needed change. However, for the rest of us, strap in, get your pen and paper handy and get ready to experience an incredible mental shift that will change the way you see, hear and feel about your future!

How many of us now are in careers, jobs or schools where we literally have no idea how we got there? We sit in our cars, stuck in traffic on the way to and from work, or maybe we stare into our computer screens wondering, "Where did I go wrong?

How did I end up here? What happened to the last five to ten years of my life?" Some of us are even performing jobs that go against everything we believe in at the very core of who we are. We may be the lawyer who wakes up every morning and dreads going into the office to meet his next client who may cause him to go against his conscience yet again in order to represent them. We may be the state worker who knows deep down that her talents are being wasted and that her fourteen-year-old daughter could do this job with her eyes closed, but yet she loves the benefits and job security. We may be the young dentist who left school with over $200,000 worth of debt and has to work on patients who really don't need the amount of dental work recommended, but who doesn't say anything because his patients were sold the extra services by the "commission enticed" office manager. Or maybe we are the pharmaceutical rep who pushes our company's latest drugs to our database of doctors even though we are very health conscious ourselves and would never even think of putting those substances in our or any of our family members' bodies. Or perhaps we are the car salesman who gets handsomely rewarded by getting clients to pay the highest amount possible for their vehicle, etc.

I am not saying this is everybody or even the majority of the people out there but you know what your own story is and what your justifications are for why you do what you do. I just want you to be aware that, if you are not currently enjoying your Dream Job mentally, physically or spiritually, the job you were designed for, the job that allows you to sleep peacefully at night, there are other options. I know this feeling personally because I have been there, many times. It didn't matter whether I was making $4 an hour or over $200,000 a year, being unhappy in your job, doing what you have to do rather than what you want to do, feeling stuck and hopeless, let's face it, really stinks! It makes you and those around you miserable, just ask my wife and kids.

In order to begin this change process, I believe it is vital to ask yourself these kinds of questions to understand where you are really at and **then** take the time to write down your answers in detail.

Why am I doing this job?

What's keeping me here even though I am miserable?

What am I really afraid of?

Why do I keep taking these types of jobs?

Is the money really worth it?

Why do I feel stuck here?

Is what I am doing glorifying my inner spiritual being?

Am I really making a difference in the world?

Is my wife happy with my career choice?

Do my kids respect my job?

If I could do anything in the world, what would I do?

Or maybe just: Why don't I have a job?

Your detailed, written answers will play a big part in helping you to determine your Obstacles and develop Strategies moving forward. I also think it's very important to ask yourself about and bring Awareness to, what kind of people you want to work with. Since you may be spending eight to twelve hours a day with these people, it's something to consider. Understand, there is a possibility that if your boss was raised in a family where he or she was never good enough, it didn't matter what they did, they were never able to please their parents, then there's a real good chance that you're going to be in a similar position where you're never going to please them and never going to be good enough either. Or, if you are surrounded in a work environment with unethical, immoral and self-gratifying co-workers, for example maybe you work in politics, (just kidding...or am I?), that will have an effect on your wellbeing too.

The reason it is so important to ask and answer these questions is because it has been said that your brain works in only three processes: the "thinking", the "doing" and the "being". (I briefly talked about this in the opening chapter). So it's important to first learn to spend the majority of your time in the thinking process: asking the right questions, seeing, hearing and feeling the 'who', the 'what', the 'when', the 'where' and the 'why' of the job you seek. Think about the small details like who you want to be working with, what kind of atmosphere you prefer to work in, why you are doing what you do, where exactly you are working and what it looks like when you walk in the front door.

You may be thinking, "how in the world will I know all that?" For example, "I don't have a choice about who my boss/manager is!" Really? You don't? I understand you could feel that way now but what if you had a New Belief that you actually do have a choice and your choice does matter and you could control that and, you don't have to be in that kind of work environment if you don't want to be. Instead, it can be your New Belief about yourself, your perfect Dream Job, the people you work with, the environment and what you believe to be true that will empower you to make that change, today! I suggest you try spending some time with those kind of thoughts and then see how you feel afterwards.

Moving past the past:

In order for this or any change to happen in your life, you MUST first get rid of the victim mindset! Because every victim needs a rescuer. You can keep screaming for help all you want but, until you change the victim mindset, you are relying on someone else (human that is) to come rescue you. And, as I am sure you are beginning to see, you are running out of people who hear your screams. How can you facilitate a lasting change in your life if you need a rescuer to help you every time? Everything in this chapter is about teaching you, empowering you and giving you the tools to make these needed changes yourself. If you choose (because really... it is only your choice) to hold onto the victim mindset, I am telling you point blank, you have already neutralized any chance of a change in this process.

Here is what the victim (excuse) mindset looks, sounds or feels like:

- If I change my major, my parents will disown me.
- I am miserable, but if I leave, my boss would be stuck without me.

- I only work here because it makes my Dad happy.
- My boss has been telling me for five years he would promote me.
- I know it doesn't feel right doing what I do, but I have no choice.
- What if I get hired and can't do the job well enough?
- I know I have the technical skills just not the people skills.
- I don't want to have to start all over again.
- Why would they ever hire me?
- I hate getting up early in the morning.
- I would have to have more training before I could get that job.
- I can't see myself taking that chance.
- What would my friends say if I did that?
- It just sounds like too much work.
- Etc.

Striving towards what's ahead:

Don't be too **discouraged** if you see any of those issues in your life or those sound like things you have said or if you have felt that way before. That is all in the past! Today is a new day! If this victim mindset has been a major road block for you, there is hope. I would suggest you go back to Chapter One and test to see if there are not some personal growth changes you need to make first. That important step will only help make this "Dream Job" change that much more effective.

There is something else I have discovered over the years of meeting with **clients**. If you have ever been fired or let go from a job, I want you to think about this: you always get what you create and you are always creating. So, as you look back to when you lost that job, be honest with yourself before you start telling me that you haven't always got what you've wanted because I am here to show you that you've always got exactly what you called forth in your beliefs. There is a good possibility, in one or two of those past instances, that you saw yourself as the "victim" on that past occasion when you lost your job. Yet, the truth is that you no longer chose that job; you stopped getting up in the morning with enthusiasm and began getting up with dread. You stopped feeling happy about going to work and began feeling resentment. You even began fantasizing about doing something else. You think these thoughts mean nothing? You misunderstand the power of your thoughts. Your life mimics your true beliefs, it can't help it. Change your beliefs, change your life!

Lastly, I would like to address and bring awareness to the fact that our world has programmed us to believe that our jobs, work, careers are more about competition then cooperation meaning, we are programmed in such a way from childhood that we must **perform** on a higher level than our co-workers or classmates in order to advance or get ahead. Take a minute here to really digest that thought. I personally have no idea when this way of thinking actually began to be implemented into our society but, from what I have seen, it is a worldwide problem. The good news is, it does not have to continue. There are a small number of cultures in remote places on this planet where this competition over cooperation does not yet exist. I have watched several documentaries on tribes and cultures where cooperation is embedded in every part of their lives. In these communities, the older more experienced members spend their whole lives helping to mentor the younger generation about how to do almost everything. Boys at a very young age are taught everything they need to become responsible providers and even young fathers, some by the age of fourteen. Girls are taught to become the "Jill of all trades" from the time they can walk and speak. The community works and succeeds only through cooperation, knowing that the benefits will enhance not only the lives of the individual but also the lives of all who presently are and will be a future part of that community.

Personally, for me, it's been rather disheartening to see how most countries nowadays are raising their future generations. Competition starts early. In school, the kids with the best grades are rewarded and celebrated, children with the best talents are made to become idols and set as examples for other kids to follow. Parents now feel the pressure for their children to succeed in everything from athletics to academics and even the new coveted "social media" life. I am not saying all this is wrong I agree we should teach our children to be the best that they can be and that we should have high expectations. I just want you to ask yourself (if you're a parent), "What is my motivation behind this?", and then spend some time thinking about the way you were raised and the expectations that were imposed on you. Were they helpful or damaging? Were you able to pursue your dreams or were you forced to become what your parents, (or whomever was the main influence in your life), dreamed for you? Did they pass down to you some of the same dysfunction their parents had passed down to them? The whole time you told yourself, "I will never be like that with my children!", yet you have not taken the time to look in the mirror and see for yourself if, presently, that is truly the case? I only bring all of this up to enhance the fact that any lasting life change can only begin with complete and detailed awareness of where you are now. So spending some time in self-reflection on why you are where you are at in this particular career stage of your life, or lack of career stage, will only help you benefit from the "Define and Find your Dream Job" process you are about to learn.

Define and Find Your Dream Job

Ok, so I know I may have **rambled** on a little to get to this point but, as with everything you read in life, take what applies to you and dump the rest. So, what do you need to do next? Think of Google maps. You can't just open the program and it guesses where you want to go. No... it's up to you to put in a specific address then it will take you there by the fastest, shortest route available. Well that is the exact goal of this "30-Minute Change" process you are about to experience to find you the perfect job. With this short exercise, you will be able to pinpoint your Dream Job and actually make it attainable in the next few days, weeks or months. You will be creating new connections in your brain by spending most of your time in the "thinking" stage. Then, when you are finished, you will start the "doing" so that you will end up in the "being", i.e. living out what you have already created in your subconscious mind.

Awareness + Obstacle + Strategy + Execution = Desired Result.

Again, we always start any desired change with personal Awareness, (if it is someone else's awareness that you need to change jobs or careers, it won't have the same effect). **Awareness** may begin with something like this: I am not in my perfect job or I need a new job or I hate my job or I just need a job and the **Obstacles** may sound something like this: I am not even sure what that job would look like for me or, I don't know how to make the transition from my comfortable job to my perfect/dream job or, I don't know where to start or, I don't believe I can do it myself or, I am afraid to make a change or, what if I fail?

Once you have personally and clearly defined your Obstacles to your Awareness, then you can move on to the next steps which is where the real transformation for this change process will begin. Before we get there, let's look at a few examples of just the **Awareness** and **Obstacles** part of the process.

1. Mary has been working at the same Law Firm as a paralegal for twelve years. It was a job she stumbled into out of college when she needed to earn enough money to get her own place in the city. She told herself it would just be a short-term job and that after two or three years she would go back to finding a job related to her major, which was

Music Appreciation. After procrastinating for ten years, she is finally ready to make the change.

THE AWARENESS: (MUST BE PERSONAL AND DETAILED.)

I don't like going to work anymore. I feel trapped in a job I can't stand.

THE OBSTACLE: (MUST BE CLEARLY DETAILED AND DEFINED.)

I don't know where to start. I am not sure what I want to do next. I have a lot of expenses. I may have to sell my condo and move to a smaller town.

2. Peter works as a manager at a large pet store chain. He started as a stock boy eight years ago and worked his way up to manager after three years. He has a secure job and likes the benefits but his passion and dream has always been to run his own business. He has had numerous opportunities to take the leap of faith and go out on his own but, whenever he is close, his fear takes over and he stays with the sure thing, the secure job.

THE AWARENESS: (MUST BE PERSONAL AND DETAILED.)

I am not being fair to the company. They want me to move to the next level of management and I keep making excuses because deep down, I want to leave tomorrow and start my own business. I need to do this for my mental wellbeing.

THE OBSTACLE: (MUST BE CLEARLY DETAILED AND DEFINED.)

The company will be disappointed in me. I have not gone to the bank to see about a small business loan. I have not completed my business plan. Even though my wife has been encouraging me to do this, I don't want to let her down. Truthfully, I am very comfortable and have a lot of control at the store.

3. Michael is a pro basketball player. He has been traveling around Europe for the last seven years playing on two

different teams. He makes a ton of money and enjoys the freedom. He has seen the world and has never had what he calls a real job, going from High School to a full ride in College to the international basketball league. As he just turned thirty, he is beginning to realize he wants to settle down. He has a few options to make it on an NBA team back in the States if he has one more good season but, deep down, he really just wants to be a barber and own his own shop. When he tells his friends they always laugh and tease him. His best memories as a kid growing up on the streets were hanging out at the barber shop and listening to the old guys tell their stories.

THE AWARENESS: (MUST BE PERSONAL AND DETAILED.)

I have accomplished everything I need to in my sport. I do not love the game like I used to. The money does not matter to me. Doing what I love and helping kids in the city is what I need to be doing now!

THE OBSTACLE: (MUST BE CLEARLY DETAILED AND DEFINED.)

My agent will try to talk me out of retiring and remind me I will be walking away from millions. My girlfriend may not choose to come along for this ride. I will have to start from scratch. I have never been a businessman.

Moving on to "The Strategy"

This will be the foundation for your dream job and can change the direction of your life forever. Even as I write this, I am overwhelmed by the excitement of how well this exercise works. I have never see a more effective interactive process to help a person define and work towards attaining their Dream Job in my life. I highly suggest you just read through the rest of the chapter first to get the gist of how the process works. Then go back, grab your notebook or if you would like to download the six-page formatted "Job Change Process" form, it is available for download now at: www.**30MinuteChange.com**

Let's begin

Assuming you have already clarified and written down your new Awareness and your Obstacles, the next thing I want you to do is list all the jobs you will not fall back on or ever want to have to do again. You know these jobs, they are always there as a default, a safety net, a sure thing - the job you can do in your sleep. This is an important exercise because it will remind you that these are no longer options in your life and they have kept you from achieving your dream job. Yes, they pay the bills and you are good at them but they lead nowhere and will not give you the desires of your heart. Maybe you're a waiter who wants to be an artist. You always start to make the transition but seem to fall back to the safe money that waiting tables brings. Or you're the salesperson who desires to go back to school to become a teacher. The dream is nice but how can you make that dream a reality with all the responsibilities you have. Or maybe you're the corporate robot who knows how to play the game very well but who secretly wants to open your own garden nursery.

After you spend a few moments thinking and writing down the jobs you won't do, next I want you to write down the job or jobs that you would love to do, dream of doing, believe to be your perfect fit, or the job you know you want to do but are afraid to do.

For this next example of the process we will be using Peter from above.

STRATEGY: STEP 1

LIST THE JOBS YOU WILL NOT FALL BACK ON OR EVER WANT TO DO AGAIN.

1. *Being a store manager*
2. *Working in retail*
3. *Working for a large Corporation*

LIST YOUR PERFECT DREAM JOBS. WHAT YOU WOULD DO IF NOTHING STOOD IN YOUR WAY.

1. *Run my own car retailing business*
2. *Buy cars at auction to resell them*
3. *Buy into a used car dealership*
4. *Start a blog on used cars*

STRATEGY: STEP 2

Now look at those three to five dream jobs and narrow it down to only two. We will only focus here on two. Pick two that you could actually do if given the opportunity. Don't say doctor if you've never been to medical school, or rock star if you can't sing. Be true to yourself. Take time to think about your talents and skills. What is unique about you, what you are good at doing? What have others told you that you would be good at doing? Here you will break down your two choices and write out all the Pros and Cons of each particular job.

DREAM JOB # 1: *Run Car Detailing Business*

Pick the two best job options from the previous sheet. Write the first one above. Take your time and find as many Pros and Cons that will accompany this job choice.

Pros of This Job:	*Cons of This Job:*
1. Be my own boss	*1. Have employees*
2. I love working on cars	*2. Liabilities & Insurances*
3. Hire my friend Jeff	*3.*
4. Flexible schedule	*4.*
5. Meet like-minded people	*5.*
6. My cars will always look nice	*6.*
7. Unlimited clients	*7.*
8. Get corporate accounts	*8.*
9. Minimal investment	*9.*
10. Able to work outside	*10.*
11. Can incorporate mobile service	*11.*
12. I have contacts for products	*12.*
13. Heavy word of mouth advertising	*13.*
14. I can mentor young men	*14.*
15.	*15.*

DREAM JOB # 2: *Start Buying Cars At Auction To Resell Them*

Pick the two best job options from the previous sheet. Write the Second one above. Take your time and find as many Pros and Cons that will accompany this job choice.

Pros of This Job	*Cons of This Job*
1. Be my own boss	*1. Could buy a lemon*
2. Make good money on the right cars	*2. Liabilities & Insurances*
3. Keep the cars I like	*3. Have to store the cars*
4. Flexible schedule	*4. Need a resale license*
5. Spend time with friends	*5. Supply may vary*
6. Get to search out deals	*6. Need to buy a tow truck*
7. Minimal investment	*7. Need a good mechanic*
8.	*8.*
9.	*9.*
10.	*10.*

Pros of This Job	Cons of This Job
11.	11.
12.	12.
13.	13.
14	14.
15.	15.

Now look over the two sheets you have filled out and pick the **one** job/career that looks, sounds and feels like the best fit for you at this time. Let your answers and thoughts about each option act as your guide to pick the perfect dream job about which to create your "New Belief".

STRATEGY: STEP 3

Here you will create your *"NEW BELIEF" statement about your newly defined "DREAM JOB".*

Dream Job you picked:

OWN AND RUN A CAR DETAILING BUSINESS.

What does your new "DREAM JOB" look, sound and feel like?

Take a moment and close your eyes. Picture yourself already working and experiencing this new dream job.
Then describe in detail what you see, hear and feel.

Visual (I see...)

- *I see myself waking up and checking my email to find ten new orders for service*
- *I see the shop I will move into. It has two large bay doors and room for six cars*
- *I see my five-star Yelp reviews growing each month*

Auditory (I hear...)

- *I hear my clients telling me how happy they are with our service*
- *I hear the sounds of a bustling shop with workers and clients*

talking together
- *I hear my phone ringing off the hook so much that I have to hire a receptionist*

Kinesthetic (I feel...)

- *I feel Excited*
- *I feel motivated*
- *I feel happy*

Now that you have seen, heard and felt what this new job will be like for you, claim it in your New Belief statement below.

Here are a few examples:

Example 1: *I am a successful finish carpenter building custom cabinets in Beverly Hills homes!*

Example 2: *I love going to the gym every day to train my committed and likeable clients.*

Example 3: *I love my job programming software for XYZ (Fortune 100) company in the Silicon Valley of sunny California.*

Example 4: *I jump out of bed every morning and walk to work at (XYZ company) where my peers respect me and treat me fairly*

YOUR NEW BELIEF STATEMENT: (ABOUT YOUR NEW DREAM JOB. MUST BE WRITTEN IN THE PRESENT TENSE)

I gratefully own and run one of the most successful auto detailing businesses in Atlanta.

WHOLE-BRAIN PROGRAMING: (THIS ADDS THE NEW BELIEF TO YOUR SUBCONSCIOUS.)

Get into a Whole-Brain Posture (sitting on a chair, legs and arms crossed).
Close your eyes and think about your new desired result belief statement.
Concentrate on experiencing a mental, emotional or physical change in your mind and body about your New Belief statement

65

as you repeat it over and over again silently.

"*I gratefully own and run one of the most successful auto detailing business in Atlanta.*"

After a few minutes you will feel a change in your thoughts, feelings or emotions.
Then open your eyes, uncross your body and Lock in the New Belief.

See appendix A in the back of this book for the detailed process of how to do the "Whole-Brain Programing" exercise.

THE EXECUTION OF YOUR DESIRED RESULT. (YOUR DREAM JOB)

This is what you tell everyone you know and meet about your perfect, DREAM JOB. The more detailed you can make this, the more opportunities there will be for others to help you.
You will only apply to jobs and to companies that meet your Desired Result. You will immediately update all your resumes and social media networks to include your "New Execution Statement".

This will be your "New Belief Statement" and "Desired result" rolled into one. So, when someone says to you, "Hey I heard you were looking for a new job!", or, "What kind of job are you looking for?, you respond.

Example 1:

I am glad you asked! The dream job I am looking for is to be a Tennessee Walker horse trainer. I want to work in the San Diego area and live on the property where I work. I want to be able to not only train horses but be able to start raising my own horses as well to sell to my clients. I want the owners of the property to work with me to build one of the top-rated training facilities in Southern California.

Example 2:

Thanks for asking, let me tell you about my perfect job. I want to work for a Fortune 500 company as a systems analyst. I want to be able to take the train to work and have my weekends off. I want to work for a young and upcoming company that believes in giving back to the environment. I want to be able to grow within the company and have the opportunity to become a team leader within the first year.

Your Final Dream Job Statement:

I have just started my own business. I have always dreamed of running a value added, high quality car detailing company that builds its reputation from quality service and satisfied clients. My company will travel as far as two hours from downtown to service my clients. My #1 goal is to be able to serve my clients and their friends and build a referral based business. Do you know anyone who is looking to get their car detailed that I could call?

Why and how this works

Now the Execution: Every action creates a reaction! So go out and tell everyone, and I mean everyone, what you want, what your perfect Dream Job is and let the energy of the universe align with you to receive it. I call this the Rifle & Shotgun approach. You use the laser focus of a rifle to define what your perfect Dream Job is, then use the shotgun to spread the word. Tell everybody, ten, twenty, one hundred or even one thousand people specifically about the Dream Job you are looking for. Let everyone work together to help you. That is why it is so important that you are very specific and clearly defined. This makes it much easier for everyone to help you.

Let me show you what this looks or sounds like:

"Hey Jim, what's up?
Not much, just looking for a new job
Oh yeah, doing what?

I don't really care, whatever, I just need a different job.
Ok man, good luck and see you later."
Or this:
"Hey Jim, what's up?
Not too much, I am just really fired up about the perfect job I am
seeking out.
Oh yeah, tell me about it.
You know how I really love animals?
Yeah
So, I am looking to work for a dog groomer as an assistant, I can
work as many hours as needed so I can learn every part of the
business while I help serve the clients. Then I am going to start my
own business next year.
Really? You know...I think my wife has a good friend who is a dog
groomer. I can give you a call later with her #.
Thanks that would be awesome."

Another example:

"Hey Tina long time no see.
Are you still working at Com-EDU doing programming?
Yes...but I hate it. Long hours and the pay is stagnant.
Bummer, any ideas on a new job?
Well I post my resume and check LinkedIn all the time but nothing
yet.
Okay well good seeing you"
Or this:
"Hey Tina long time no see.
Are you still working at Com-EDU doing programming?
Yes...but I am not very happy there. Long hours and the pay is
stagnant.
Bummer, any ideas on a new job?
I am glad you asked, as a matter of fact I am really excited about my
dream job. I am looking to get on with a startup, preferably one in
the medical field. I really see myself working for a company that is
on the cutting edge of new medical technology. I want to be less than
thirty minutes from my home and get paid for my skills.
Well Tina, now that you mention it. I am part of a network of young
entrepreneurs. I know many of them are in the medical field. Why
don't you come to a meeting with me this Thursday and see if you
can make some contacts?"

Another example:

Facebook/LinkedIn post:
Hey everyone! I am making an exciting change in my life right now and would really love your help. I have defined my dream job and want to share it with you and am asking for any help or suggestions you may have in helping me attain my Dream Job:
Let me tell you about it. I want to be working in the parks and recreation department in or near Sacramento which will allow me the honor of beautifying the surrounding areas and providing a safe environment for children, families and people in general. It also provides an opportunity to get to know people and share my faith. It can be for the city, state or even a college. I want to work full time and have my weekends off.

The power of getting others involved:

I believe we were created to help each other with this thing called life. As the great prophet Jesus Christ once said, "There is no greater gift than to lay down one's life for a friend."

Doing something for someone else is how we are able to keep in touch with our **heart**, that powerful force that is only strengthened by loving and unconditional giving to others. I also believe that when you ask for something with pure motives, the invisible energy forces that operate behind the scenes at the Quantum level, adjust to give you exactly what you ask for. When you take the time to align your true self with your desired purpose and then humbly ask others for help...watch what happens!

Imagine being a business owner and having everyone who works for you working in their respective "Dream Job". It doesn't matter if they are the janitor, the secretary, the accountant or the CEO as long as they are working in the exact job they had defined and set their New Belief to. What kind of a company would that be! As opposed to having people who work for you wishing they were doing something else.

I want you to believe that if you take the time to work through this exercise and clearly define your Dream Job, then begin to let everyone know what it is, there is absolutely no doubt you will find that opportunity, because others will bring it to you. We all know how hard it is to help people who do not know that they need help or what help they need. Our intentions may be good but it takes a willing party on the other side. Let us not be those people! Let our New Belief clearly define our "Dream Job Statement".

Even now, your emotions may want to overwhelm you. You know you need to make a career change, start a business, leave something that you know is harmful, etc. and that is where you have been stuck in the past. What if you could change your belief to be one that "knew" if you would just ask for help and guidance, it would be there for you at any time. If you spent enough time empowering your thoughts in the Awareness and thinking stage rather than the default "limiting programmed emotional stage" you are so comfortable in, would you not then be able to clearly see the help you needed?

There is a reason you are reading this chapter, in this book, at this present time on your journey. It is not by accident. So, with that new Awareness, it's up to you to create a New Belief about your Dream Job by re-reading this chapter, grabbing your notebook, or downloading the process change forms at **www.The30MinuteChange.com** or I suggest signing up for a onetime life changing coaching session to help guide you through this step toward your Dream Job.

Chapter 3

Relationships

"We do not walk backwards to get to where we want to go.
So why don't we stop thinking backwards and become who we want to be."

Here is a Facebook post from my friend Jenn who, six months earlier, lost her firefighter husband while he was on duty, leaving her widowed with two young children:

"I wish I could say that our marriage was flawless but, the truth is, we worked crazy hard for it. It took time to learn how to be the kind of wife he deserved and it took him time to learn how to be the communicator I needed. Want to know when our marriage changed and we became the happiest we had ever been? When I stopped waiting for him to change. Prior to his passing I had been asked how we changed our marriage. My answer every time: 'break the cycle.' It takes humility to be the one to break the cycle. It means swallowing pride. It means accepting faults. It means loving without expectation. We stared divorce in the face. As God would have it, He moved things around and brought Ryan and I back together. But we still didn't have it right. There was no big meeting between us. There was no declaration that we were going to change. I

recognized my faults as a wife (Awareness), I acknowledged the areas I could change (Obstacle) and I did it. I changed my perspective (Strategy). Instead of waiting for him to change, I noticed everything that already made him great (Execution). Ryan felt a huge change IN me. So that made him change FOR me (Desired Result). The cycle was broken. I could've waited. I could've said, 'no way. He's the one who needs to change.' If I would've waited, well, I hate to think about the regrets I would have now. I have no regrets. My only regret is that I didn't break the cycle early in our marriage. Are you stuck in your marriage/relationship? Break the cycle. Stop waiting for him/her to change. Be the one to change and then watch what happens. You're not 'giving in' when you break the cycle. You're not "weak." Humility takes great strength. Think about it: if there's a boulder in your way, what do you do? Do you just stare at it because you're afraid that moving it will hurt? Or do you give it everything you have to push that thing out of the way so you can get to your destination? It may hurt, you may be exhausted, but when you look back and see that boulder you moved, you'll find the strength to move another."

These are her words exactly as she posted them. I just added the AOSED process in parentheses. Jenn has never read my book nor have I ever discussed the "30 Minute Change" with her but you can see the conscious step by step process she went through to make the desired change. Just as I have talked about earlier in this book, the AOSED process is naturally hard wired into all of us. Which means it is accessible to us anytime we need it. Yes, it can take time to discover, time to clarify, time to see the need to change, etc. but what I am hoping to bring to your Awareness as you read through this book, is that the change process can indeed happen sooner rather than later, by bringing to your attention the need to change and giving you back the power and tools to initiate that change. Today!

Being married myself for over twenty-nine years now, I have learned a few things; most of these came out of trial and error, meaning I tried and my wife pointed out my error. I'm just kidding! Most of my growth came out of the Awareness that I had no idea what I was doing and needed to seek loads of help. When I say seek loads of help, I mean seeking it from people who were successful at it, not what you see on "The Real Housewives of _____". I remember very early in our marriage, we were maybe twenty-three, we had two kids, I was a struggling actor/waiter and we were barely scraping by. We were too broke to afford to pay to see a counsellor so we found a free service through a local church. We met with this really quirky single guy who said he had never dated and who still lived with his mother - we met in his kitchen in West LA. After walking out of there, I remember my wife and I looking at each other laughing and thinking, "oh my gosh, maybe we are not that bad off after all." So, we walked away realizing we needed to find more help, maybe some other couples who were working to have a good marriage and imitate what they were doing.

The truth is, I do not think there is anything more challenging in our lives than relationships. We were conceived through a relationship, born into a relationship, raised in many different types of relationships and will spend the rest of our waking moments fumbling through various relationships. How helpful would it be if we could learn how to get better at them sooner, rather than later? One way I have found to help is by bringing clarity to the relationship and taking the time to separate the emotions from the facts.

Facts versus emotions. Let me start by reminding you again of the importance of asking yourself questions first. What does the word "fact" mean to you? What does the word "emotion" mean to you? I want to briefly talk about these two subjects because I believe it will help you tremendously as you work through many different types of relationships in your life. By bringing awareness to the extreme differences of these two thought patterns, facts versus emotions, you will gain the tools required to turn the lights on in many dark and ugly situations.

What is a fact? The dictionary defines it as: something that actually exists, reality, truth. Something that has already happened.

What is emotion? The dictionary defines it as: any strong agitation of the feelings activated by experiencing love, hate, fear, etc., and usually accompanied by certain physiological changes, as increased heartbeat or respiration, and often overt manifestation, as crying or shaking. Many times, lasting only a short moment.

Ok... so to overly simplify it. A fact is true and an emotion is a brief feeling we may have.

Let's see what I am talking about with a few examples:

Todd and Keith, best friends for eighteen years. They met in the first grade and have been friends ever since. They went to the same schools, played the same sports and their families went on vacation together. Todd graduated from college and has a high paying job. Keith left school a year early to help his mom after his father passed away. Todd was there for Keith a lot during the first few months but his new job has him flying all over and keeps him very busy. Keith believes Todd is too good for him now because he is making great money, has a new car and a hot girlfriend. In his mind, Todd has changed and is no longer a good friend. He has decided to forget about him and not call him anymore to hang out.

Facts: Todd has a new job that keeps him busy. He has a new girlfriend because that brings him joy. He can afford a new car. He still cares for Keith and considers him a best friend.

Emotions: Keith feels left out and he's a little jealous. He is still struggling after his father's death. He feels hurt by Todd because he is not spending as much time with him anymore. To protect himself, he is going to cut Todd out of his life.

All of this is going on inside of Keith and he is not aware of the reasons behind any of it. He just wants it to stop, so he makes a rash decision that he thinks will ease the pain.

Alicia has been married to **Jeffrey** for ten years. They have two kids and Jeffrey has had trouble keeping a job ever since they met. Alicia works full time, does most of the cooking and helps the kids with homework and chores. Alicia loves Jeffrey so she puts up with all his faults. Jeffrey stays out late most nights and has a drinking problem. Alicia is aware of at least two affairs he has had but has been afraid to confront Jeffrey.

Facts: Jeffrey is not being a loving partner in this marriage. He does not provide for his family and is cheating on his wife. He will not seek the help he needs. Alicia is an enabler. She thinks she loves Jeffrey, but the fact that she continues to put her head in the sand means she really doesn't love him enough to force him to face the "consequences of his choices" which, chances are, would happen if she left him. Until Jeffrey hits rock bottom, he will not change.

Emotions: Alicia is from a broken family and told herself she would never do that to her kids. She forces herself to be ok with it. She is afraid to deal with Jeffrey's issues. What will everyone think if she leaves him? The fear of change and going back on her promise to herself will keep Alicia in this terrible situation and that may end up robbing her and her children of a better life with a father who could, given the right motivation, change and come to his senses.

I bring these examples up to remind you that, if you are not careful, your emotions can and will become your beliefs. Your beliefs determine your thoughts and your behavior and ultimately the outcome of your life.

Another critical part of the relationship process is being able to love yourself first. Not in a selfish way, very few people have a problem doing that, but in a way of loving and accepting yourself as you are so knowing that you are not perfect and never will be, but recognizing that you are actively working on changing to become a better person - being able to accept your past without it being the driving force in your present. One thing I have learned after thousands of hours of coaching, mentoring and helping teens, singles and marrieds, is that we all come from dysfunctional families to one degree or another some much worse than others of course but none of us, obviously, had the choice of which family we were born into. What I have also discovered is that those who now have healthy relationships have been able to separate their dysfunctional past from their present and believe they have the ability to create a different life going forward.

One of the biggest stumbling blocks in any relationship, is forgiveness: either asking for it, giving it or accepting it from others. I call this the black hole of the heart. It darkens the perception of how one views all relationships. It is why most people cannot "give their whole heart". Even Jesus talked about being able to forgive each other from the heart, unconditional forgiveness, forgiving seven times, seventy times and not keeping a record of wrongs. For many of us that seems like a bit of a stretch. It is much easier to forgive someone in our head, i.e. they wronged us, they even said they were sorry and we understand why they did it...maybe. We accept their words but then we still harbor a bitterness, anger, fear or lack of trust in that relationship. Now times that by five, ten, twenty or one hundred different people who have done us wrong. And you wonder why relationships are such a challenge?

There are literally tens of thousands of books on relationships and forgiveness which you can read and I don't really want this to be another one. I just hope to help bring to your awareness the value of and empowerment that you can attain by studying, practicing and learning to forgive, sooner rather than later. It always has been and always will be the most important ingredient in any relationship.

Here is a list of possible relationship changes needed:

- More patience
- Express gratitude
- Gratitude
- Expressiveness
- Vulnerability
- Letting the walls down
- Focus on listening and not problem solving. (men)
- Learning to ask questions
- Seeking advice
- Forgiveness
- Controlling emotions
- Self-improvement first
- Gentleness
- Following through
- Acts of kindness

Now let's look at a few examples taken through the AOSED change process:

Example 1:

Joy is miserable. She has been dating Ken for two years. They will have a few good months and then follow that up with two or three weeks of emotional dodgeball. She knows deep down this is not the guy for her long term because they have created unhealthy, mean habits, but she is afraid to be alone. She does not have a good track record with long term relationships and doesn't know what to do. She has recently become aware, that the real problem is, she expects her boyfriends to be everything in her life, which they never will be and also, that deep down, she is unhappy with where she is at, at this stage of life. (Note: She had to go back and do a Personal Growth change before addressing the relationship change)

RELATIONSHIP CHANGE PROCESS FORM

THE AWARENESS: (MUST BE PERSONAL AND DETAILED.)

This relationship is unhealthy and I need to break it off.

THE OBSTACLE: (MUST BE CLEARLY DETAILED AND DEFINED.)

I don't want to hurt him. He will not understand the changes I need to make personally. What will I do with all my free time?

THE STRATEGY: (MUST BE THOUGHT OUT, DETAILED AND COMMITTED TO.)

Talk with him tonight and let him know where I am at. Go back to school and take some classes I am interested in. Call my old friends and apologize for not spending much time with them.

WHAT IS THE NEW BELIEF YOU WANT TO HAVE?
(THIS IS A ROUGH DRAFT THOUGHT HERE. YOU WILL CLARIFY LATER IN THE PROCESS.)

I am capable of healthy relationships with boundaries.

Pros of This Choice	Cons of This Choice
Not so much drama	*Will miss him*
More peace within	*Will be alone more*
Meet new friends	*So many good memories*
Have a social life	*Will have to tell friends*
Don't need a relationship now	
Get back in school	

Pros of This Choice	**Cons of This Choice**

Able to dream again
More time with friends
See more of my family
Better sleep
Feel empowered
Take a yoga class
My dad will be happy
Be more independent

(Take your time and write down as many Pros and Cons as you can think of! This helps solidify why this New Belief is valuable to you.)

WHAT THAT NEW STRATEGY LOOKS, SOUNDS AND FEELS LIKE.

Take a moment and close your eyes. Picture yourself already living out this New Belief.

Then describe in detail what you see, hear and feel.

Visual (I see...)

- *I see myself sitting alone on the couch reading peacefully with my cat.*
- *I see myself at the beach with the girls, laying in the sun talking and laughing.*
- *I see myself having friends over for dinner and being okay alone.*

Auditory (I hear...)

- *I hear myself telling myself, "you made the right choice."*
- *I hear my phone ring all day and it is not Ken.*
- *I hear my friend Steph telling me how much she missed spending time with me.*

Kinesthetic (I feel...)

- *I feel peaceful.*
- *I feel content.*
- *I feel very happy.*

THE EXECUTION: (MUST BE TIED TO YOUR STRATEGY AND PUT

INTO MOTION IMMEDIATELY)

Ask Ken to come over after work. Tell him what I have to do for myself. Apologize for treating him the way I have. Stand firm. Call Steph and see if I can come spend the weekend with her. On Monday register for at least two classes.

THE DESIRED RESULT: (YOUR NEW PERSONAL BELIEF STATEMENT)

I am capable of healthy relationships because I love and accept myself.

WHOLE-BRAIN PROGRAMING: (This adds the New Belief to your subconscious. Before starting this final exercise, read though your whole change process form one more time.)

Get into a Whole-Brain Posture (sitting on a chair, legs and arms crossed).
Close your eyes and think about your new desired result belief statement.
"I am capable of healthy relationships because I love and accept myself."
Concentrate on experiencing a mental, emotional or physical change in your mind and body about your new belief statement as you repeat it over and over again silently.
After a few minutes you will feel a change in your thoughts, feelings or emotions.
Then open your eyes, uncross your body and Lock in the New Belief.
See appendix A in the back of this book for the detailed process of how to do the "Whole-Brain Programing" exercise.

Example 2:

Brandon and his wife Elise have been married for sixteen years. They have two small children and both have busy jobs that keep them away from home until late hours. They were high school sweethearts and really love each other. Over the last few years, they have become distant. Their patience with each other is pretty much non-existent. They both feel like roommates and single parents, afraid that divorce may be right around the corner. They decide to attend a few marriage classes at their local place of worship. Excitingly, they become aware that their marriage and family are still the most important things to each of them. They are going to make some radical changes and they sit down together to do that. (Note: There may be times when you can do a change together but only if you are on the exact same page with regard to the change needed.)

RELATIONSHIP CHANGE PROCESS FORM

THE AWARENESS: (MUST BE PERSONAL AND DETAILED.)
We love and miss each other and want to simplify our lives.

THE OBSTACLE: (MUST BE CLEARLY DETAILED AND DEFINED.)
We both have high stress jobs. We have too much debt. We were trying to accumulate for the future but if we don't make some changes there will be no future.

THE STRATEGY: (MUST BE THOUGHT OUT, DETAILED AND COMMITTED TO.)
Brandon will ask for a raise. Elise will cut her hours to two days a week and work from home. Take kids out of childcare. Turn in one of the leased cars and pay cash for a small car. Have dinners together as a family five nights a week.

WHAT IS THE NEW BELIEF YOU WANT TO HAVE?
(THIS IS A ROUGH DRAFT THOUGHT HERE. YOU WILL CLARIFY LATER IN THE PROCESS.)
We are the most important things in each other's lives.

Pros of This Choice	Cons of This Choice
Time together with kids	*Not as much in savings*
Less stress at home	*Will miss my friends at work*
Go to the park with kids	*Live on a tight budget*

Pros of This Choice	Cons of This Choice

Live simpler
Go on dates
Fix up around the house
No more strangers raising our kids
More time with other family
Spend less eating out
We will eat healthier
Enjoy life with each other
Able to garden together
Train our children.
Have breakfast together

(Take your time and write down as many Pros and Cons as you can think of! This helps solidify why this new belief is valuable to you.)

WHAT THAT NEW STRATEGY LOOKS, SOUNDS AND FEELS LIKE.

Take a moment and close your eyes. Picture yourself already living out this New Belief.
Then describe in detail what you see, hear and feel.

Visual (I see…)

- *I see myself sitting on the bed reading my girls a story.*
- *I see myself getting dressed up to go on a date to our favorite restaurant.*
- *I see myself working on the computer as the girls play nicely in my home office.*

Auditory (I hear…)

- *I hear Brandon tell me the house looks amazing.*
- *I hear Elise telling me how the girls are always telling her about our adventures.*
- *I hear the girls laughing in the yard while we sit on the deck enjoying a glass of wine.*

Kinesthetic (I feel…)

- *I feel refreshed.*

- *I feel passionate.*
- *I feel energetic.*
- *I feel like it used to when we first dated.*

THE EXECUTION: (MUST BE TIED TO YOUR STRATEGY AND PUT INTO MOTION IMMEDIATELY)

Brandon will explain to his boss what is going on and ask for a raise. Brandon will turn in the highest leased car at the end of the month. Elise will tell her boss that she will need to give her notice and suggest they make her part time and let her work from home. Elise will let the day care know that they will be pulling the kids out after this month end. Elise will brush up on her cooking skills.

THE DESIRED RESULT: (YOUR NEW PERSONAL BELIEF STATEMENT)

Our family is more important than our future financial security.

WHOLE-BRAIN PROGRAMING: (This adds the New Belief to your subconscious. Before starting this final exercise, read though your whole change process form one more time.)

Get into a Whole-Brain Posture (sitting on a chair, legs and arms crossed).
Close your eyes and think about your new desired result belief statement.

"Our family is more important than our future financial security."

Concentrate on experiencing a mental, emotional or physical change in your mind and body about your new belief statement as you repeat it over and over again silently.
After a few minutes you will feel a change in your thoughts, feelings or emotions.
Then open your eyes, uncross your body and Lock in the New Belief.

Example 3:

Twan is successful musician. He lives in NYC and has a

busy life. He was a single child and has been estranged from his parents for many years; they basically cut him off after he dropped out of dental school and told them he was going to be a musician. He has not spoken to them in eight years and now that he is in a new relationship, he is beginning to see how this has been affecting his past relationships, specifically with regard to being able to really love someone. He is aware that his hatred for his parents is not really that, but instead a deep longing to feel accepted by them.

RELATIONSHIP CHANGE PROCESS FORM

THE AWARENESS: (MUST BE PERSONAL AND DETAILED.)
I need to reconcile with my parents.

THE OBSTACLE: (MUST BE CLEARLY DETAILED AND DEFINED.)
I have hated them for so long. I am not sure they want to see me. What if I forgive them but they don't forgive me?

THE STRATEGY: (MUST BE THOUGHT OUT, DETAILED AND COMMITTED TO.)
Let the band know I need some time off. Find out where my parents will be. Think about what I want to say. Commit to making this happen now.

WHAT IS THE NEW BELIEF YOU WANT TO HAVE?
(THIS IS A ROUGH DRAFT THOUGHT HERE. YOU WILL CLARIFY LATER IN THE PROCESS.)

My parents will be happy to see me.

Pros of This Choice:	**Cons of This Choice:**
Reconcile with parents *Feel released from my anger* *Might be told to leave* *Invite them to a show*	*May not forgive me*

Pros of This Choice:	**Cons of This Choice:**

Hugs from my mother
Play music for them
Share the last eight years of my life
Home cooked meals
They can visit me in New York
Time away from the band

(Take your time and write down as many Pros and Cons as you can think of! This helps solidify why this new belief is valuable to you.)

WHAT THAT NEW STRATEGY LOOKS, SOUNDS AND FEELS LIKE.

Take a moment and close your eyes. Picture yourself already living out this New Belief.
Then describe in detail what you see, hear and feel.

Visual (I see...)

- *I see myself sitting on the plane relaxed and calm.*
- *I see myself pulling up to the house, getting out of the cab with flowers in my hand.*
- *I see me sitting around the dinner table with my parents, eating and laughing.*

Auditory (I hear...)

- *I hear my mother tell me over and over how much she has missed me.*
- *I hear my dad asking me to play him a song.*
- *I hear my mom sing along as I play her favorite song.*

Kinesthetic (I feel...)

- *I feel complete.*
- *I feel whole.*
- *I feel loved.*

THE EXECUTION: (MUST BE TIED TO YOUR STRATEGY AND PUT INTO MOTION IMMEDIATELY)

I will call my Uncle and find out when they will be at home. Buy a plane ticket this week. Think through, write down and rehearse what I want to say. Do not hold onto one negative thought about how it will go. Stay as long as it takes to reconcile, even if it takes a month.

THE DESIRED RESULT: (YOUR NEW PERSONAL BELIEF STATEMENT)

I am loved and accepted by my family just the way I am.

WHOLE-BRAIN PROGRAMING: (This adds the New Belief to your subconscious. Before starting this final exercise, read though your whole change process form one more time.)

Get into a Whole-Brain Posture (sitting on a chair, legs and arms crossed).
Close your eyes and think about your new desired result belief statement.

"I am loved and accepted by my family just the way I am."

Concentrate on experiencing a mental, emotional or physical change in your mind and body about your new belief statement as you repeat it over and over again silently.
After a few minutes you will feel a change in your thoughts, feelings or emotions.
Then open your eyes, uncross your body and Lock in the New Belief.

There will always be changes to make in our relationships as they are ever evolving. Here are some other examples of possible needed changes.

- I want to do special things for her
- Plan a vacation
- Once a week date nights
- Take a class together
- Write him special notes before work
- Call my mom once a week

- Find my son and go see him
- Forgive my sister and then call her
- Write my father a letter and place it on his grave.
- Be the first to apologize
- Etc....

As much as we sometimes try to convince ourselves that we are better off alone, the fact is, we were never meant to be alone. Relationships with the right beliefs can be the most amazing and fulfilling part of our lives. We must always remember that we cannot change anyone to be what we want them to be, but we can learn to appreciate and accept them as they are.

The changes you will make by taking the time to go through one of these exercises will amaze you. You can take out a piece of paper and do this anytime you want to make a change or if you would like to download a set of "Change Process" forms that are already created for you to just fill in, they are available for download at: **www30MinuteChange.com**

Chapter 4

New Hobbies

*"There is no greater power than the power of choice.
There is no greater choice than to choose to control that power."*

I realize that this is a chapter you would not normally see in a self-improvement book but I hope to help make you *aware* of how important and empowering hobbies can be in your life. For many of you, your childhood completely revolved around hobbies - playing with toys, dolls, Lego, video games, riding bikes, shooting hoops, jumping rope, playing organized sports, dance or art classes, etc... Work was just something your parents did. You, on the other hand, spent most of your time playing. Yes, you had to go to school for six or seven hours a day but when you got home, it was play time. Now, as adults, many of you have brought your childhood memories of "adults just work" into your belief system. While it is true, very true, that you have more responsibilities now as an adult than you had as a kid, it doesn't mean that when you get home you can't or shouldn't have play time. I would like you to stop reading here for a few minutes and take some time to reflect on some of the fun things you spent time doing when you were younger. Close your eyes and focus on seeing yourself doing those things now.

"Meditation Pause Here"

That was nice huh? As children we did not have to be told to "be here now", it was natural for us to be totally engaged in what we were doing at the time, i.e. living in the moment. When I was playing in a neighborhood game of football in the vacant lot across the street, I was not thinking about all the homework I had do the next day. When I was playing Monopoly with my sisters, I was not thinking about how I needed to clean my room before dinner. Hobbies were and still need to be our escape, the things we do to keep our minds off the things we have to do. Because of the ease in which we can "veg out" in front of the TV, computer or phone, hobbies are becoming less and less a part of the lives of the younger generations. When I was growing up, there was no reason to be inside. If you were inside there was a good chance you would be asked to do a chore or told to go and read a book. Because of the lack of electronics, we were forced to find or create new things to do. Boredom brought about many new creative things to do; if you look back to the beginning of time, that was how hobbies came to be.

How does that saying go? "All work and no play makes Jack a sad sack", or something along those lines. I hope you have realized by this time in your life that the world is pretty much a "work = reward" based system and it always has been. I am not here to judge whether it is fair or not, I am just stating the facts. If you don't believe this, spend some time remembering your childhood, looking at the school systems, analyzing any company in the world or observing how animals are trained etc... Work = Reward!

So, let's spend time in this chapter helping you make some awesome changes that will help you reward yourself for all your hard work.

Example 1:

Jane knows all she does is work and take care of her family. She believes there is no way she will have enough time to add a new hobby to the overwhelming schedule she has now. She desperately wants to be able to get back into ballet or some form of dancing. She remembers how much she enjoyed it and how it helps relieve stress.

NEW HOBBIES CHANGE PROCESS FORM

THE AWARENESS: (MUST BE PERSONAL AND DETAILED.)

I need to make time to do something for myself, like take a dance class.

THE OBSTACLE: (MUST BE CLEARLY DETAILED AND DEFINED.)

I work long hours. The kids' schedules are demanding. My husband travels quite a bit. There is no available night. Maybe I don't really want to do it bad enough!

THE STRATEGY: (MUST BE THOUGHT OUT, DETAILED AND COMMITTED TO.)

Rethink my priorities around the kids' schedule. Cut my hours at work. Find a class I am interested in taking.

WHAT IS THE NEW BELIEF YOU WANT TO HAVE? (THIS IS A ROUGH DRAFT THOUGHT HERE. YOU WILL CLARIFY LATER IN THE PROCESS.)

I find time to do the things that I love to do.

Pros of This Choice	**Cons of This Choice**
I will be more joyful	*Rework schedule again*
I will be less stressed	*Have to be on a budget*
My kids will complain	
I will feel better physically	
Work will be less consuming	
I will feel more at peace	
I will meet new people outside work	
I love to dance	
I can be as free as a little girl again	
My husband will be glad I am doing this for myself	
I will have time to myself	

(Take your time and write down as many Pros and Cons as you can think of! This helps solidify why this New Belief is valuable to you.)

WHAT THAT NEW STRATEGY LOOKS, SOUNDS AND FEELS LIKE.

Take a moment and close your eyes. Picture yourself already living out this New Belief.
Then describe in detail what you see, hear and feel.

Visual (I see...)

- *I see myself looking into the mirror dressed in my light pink leotard.*
- *I see my husband and kids sitting in the audience watching my performance.*
- *I see myself sitting on the floor in class stretching to peaceful music.*

Auditory (I hear...)

- *I hear my husband telling me he is very proud of me.*
- *I hear my daughter Katie telling me how good I look in my outfit.*
- *I hear my teacher telling me "I can see you have been dancing for years."*

Kinesthetic (I feel...)

- *I feel young again.*
- *I feel firm and can feel my muscles.*
- *I feel peaceful.*

THE EXECUTION: (MUST BE TIED TO YOUR STRATEGY AND PUT INTO MOTION IMMEDIATELY)

I will talk with my kids and let them know they have to drop one of their three activities. I will talk to my boss about leaving early one day a week. I will go online tonight and find an eight to twelve week dance class and sign up.

THE DESIRED RESULT: (YOUR NEW PERSONAL BELIEF STATEMENT.)

I joyfully and consciously make time to do things that are important to me.

WHOLE-BRAIN PROGRAMING: (This adds the New Belief to your subconscious. Before starting this final exercise, read though your whole change process form one more time.)

Get into a Whole-Brain Posture (sitting on a chair, legs and arms crossed).
Close your eyes and think about your new desired result belief statement.

"I joyfully and consciously make time to do things that are important to me."

Concentrate on experiencing a mental, emotional or physical change in your mind and body about your New Belief statement as you repeat it over and over again silently.
After a few minutes you will feel a change in your thoughts, feelings or emotions.
Then open your eyes, uncross your body and Lock in the New Belief.

See appendix A in the back of this book for the detailed process of how to do the "Whole-Brain Programing" exercise.

Example 2:

Nicholas is a commission only salesman. He has been with his current company for six years now. With all of his success, he still works weekends and never turns off his phone. For the last three years, he has been talking about getting his pilot's license but always has an excuse as to why "it's not the right time". He is ready to make a change.

NEW HOBBIES CHANGE PROCESS FORM

THE AWARENESS: (MUST BE PERSONAL AND DETAILED.)

I need to get my pilot's license!

THE OBSTACLE: (MUST BE CLEARLY DETAILED AND DEFINED.)

I love my job and being the #1 sales guy. If I take my eye off the ball I may drop below my expectations. I will have to study to pass the test and I am not good at tests.

THE STRATEGY: (MUST BE THOUGHT OUT, DETAILED AND COMMITTED TO.)

Look online for flight schools. Set aside time to accomplish this goal. Start studying for the test now.

WHAT IS THE NEW BELIEF YOU WANT TO HAVE?
(THIS IS A ROUGH DRAFT THOUGHT HERE. YOU WILL CLARIFY LATER IN THE PROCESS.)

I am a licensed single engine pilot.

Pros of This Choice	Cons of This Choice
I can fly to see my friends	*Have to study for hours*
I will do what I have dreamed of	*Miss time at work*
I can fly anytime I want	*May lose some deals*
I can take my girlfriend flying	
I achieved my goal	
I can escape from work	
I can buy my own plane	

Pros of This Choice	Cons of This Choice

I will see cool places from the air
I can brag to my friends
I will conquer my fear of tests
I can fly my friends around
I can disappear in the clouds

(Take your time and write down as many Pros and Cons as you can think of! This helps solidify why this New Belief is valuable to you.)

WHAT THAT NEW STRATEGY LOOKS, SOUNDS AND FEELS LIKE.

Take a moment and close your eyes. Picture yourself already living out this New Belief.

Then describe in detail what you see, hear and feel.

Visual (I see…)

- *I see myself smoothly landing the plane on the runway.*
- *I see myself opening the letter from the state saying I passed my final test.*
- *I see myself walking around my plane doing a pre-flight check.*

Auditory (I hear…)

- *I hear my instructor say "great landing!"*
- *I hear my best friend Alan telling me "Way to go bro."*
- *I hear the sound of the engine roaring during takeoff.*

Kinesthetic (I feel…)

- *I feel free. I feel powerful. I feel light.*

THE EXECUTION: (MUST BE TIED TO YOUR STRATEGY AND PUT INTO MOTION IMMEDIATELY)

Go online today and find three flight schools and set up appointments to visit them this weekend. Buy a used aviation book on Amazon. Block out in my calendar Tuesday and Thursday nights from five to eight p.m. for flight training.

THE DESIRED RESULT: (YOUR NEW PERSONAL BELIEF STATEMENT.)

I am a licensed pilot who loves flying his plane two days a week.

WHOLE-BRAIN PROGRAMING: (This adds the New Belief to your subconscious. Before starting this final exercise, read though your whole change process form one more time.)

Get into a Whole-Brain Posture (sitting on a chair, legs and arms crossed).
Close your eyes and think about your new desired result belief statement.

"I am a licensed pilot who loves flying his plane two days a week."

Concentrate on experiencing a mental, emotional or physical change in your mind and body about your New Belief statement as you repeat it over and over again silently.
After a few minutes you will feel a change in your thoughts, feelings or emotions.
Then open your eyes, uncross your body and Lock in the New Belief.

Example 3:

Franklin recently lost his wife of fifty-one years. He lives outside of town and most of his close friends have moved or passed away. He spends too much time alone and is starting to realize he needs to do something about it.

NEW HOBBIES CHANGE PROCESS FORM

THE AWARENESS: (MUST BE PERSONAL AND DETAILED.)

I need to find something to keep me busy. I need to meet some new people.

THE OBSTACLE: (MUST BE CLEARLY DETAILED AND DEFINED.)

I was married for fifty-one years and have not had to do anything alone in over thirty years. I am afraid to get out there and meet strangers. I don't know where to start.

THE STRATEGY: (MUST BE THOUGHT OUT, DETAILED AND COMMITTED TO.)

Decide on a new hobby or club to join. Get out of the house more often. Turn off the TV. Ask for help.

WHAT IS THE NEW BELIEF YOU WANT TO HAVE?
(THIS IS A ROUGH DRAFT THOUGHT HERE. YOU WILL CLARIFY LATER IN THE PROCESS.)

I can meet new people and feel comfortable

Pros of This Choice	**Cons of This Choice**
I will keep busy	*Have to get out of myself*
Meet new people	*Risk embarrassment*
Learn to take risks	
Have people to talk with	
Find a travel companion	
Get out of the house	
Learn new things	
My kids will be very happy	
Have people come visit me	
Get some exercise	

(Take your time and write down as many Pros and Cons as you can think of! This helps solidify why this New Belief is valuable to you.)

WHAT THAT NEW STRATEGY LOOKS, SOUNDS AND FEELS LIKE.

Take a moment and close your eyes. Picture yourself already living out this New Belief.
Then describe in detail what you see, hear and feel.

Visual (I see...)

- *I see myself sitting at a table with four or five guys playing cards.*
- *I see myself learning to send and receive emails.*
- *I see myself playing golf with a new set of friends.*

Auditory (I hear...)

- *I hear my wife telling me in a dream to get out there and do it.*
- *I hear my daughter laughing over the phone after I tell her about the class I joined.*
- *I hear the busy talk of people at the senior center.*

Kinesthetic (I feel...)

- *I feel confident. I feel relaxed.*

THE EXECUTION: (MUST BE TIED TO YOUR STRATEGY AND PUT INTO MOTION IMMEDIATELY)

I will go to the senior center tomorrow and sign up for at least one class. I will get out of the house three days a week, going to the Diner, senior center or park to meet new people. I will ask my daughters if they have any ideas for my new plan. I will turn off the TV from eleven a.m. until five p.m.

THE DESIRED RESULT: (YOUR NEW PERSONAL BELIEF STATEMENT.)

I enjoy meeting new people and doing new things.

WHOLE-BRAIN PROGRAMING: (This adds the New Belief to your subconscious. Before starting this final exercise, read though your whole change process form one more time.)

Get into a Whole-Brain Posture (sitting on a chair, legs and arms crossed).
Close your eyes and think about your new desired result belief statement.

"I enjoy meeting new people and doing new things."

Concentrate on experiencing a mental, emotional or physical change in your mind and body about your new belief statement

as you repeat it over and over again silently.

After a few minutes you will feel a change in your thoughts, feelings or emotions.

Then open your eyes, uncross your body and Lock in the New Belief.

Other possible example of Awareness with regard to New Hobbies change:

- I would like to learn another language.
- I want to take up sailing.
- I need to get back into fishing.
- I would like to be a Big Brother/Big Sister.
- I want to learn how to develop an App.
- I want to learn how to play the piano.
- I want to start a blog.
- I want to start canning vegetables.
- I want to compete in Spartan races.
- I want to learn how to swing dance.
- Etc....

The changes you will make by taking the time to go through one of these exercises will amaze you. You can take out a piece of paper and do this anytime you want to make a change or if you would like to download a set of "Change Process" forms that are already created for you to just fill in, they are available for download at: **www.30MinuteChange.com**

Chapter 5

Health & Fitness

*"People ask me...'Are you really saying that a person can change anything
In their life In 30 Minutes or less?' Yes I am! If you become aware of a
Change you need to make in your Life, and you follow this detailed
Simple process, do the exercises and accept your New Belief,
You will make that change."*

What is health? What does health mean to you? What is fitness? What is the point of fitness? Why is fitness something you need in your life? Will you live a better life if you are fit and healthy? Can you be perfectly happy being unfit and unhealthy?

By honestly answering any of these questions, you may discover that those answers may not be the true motivator needed to help make the upcoming change. For example, health for you may mean being able to wake up at six a.m. and be able to get out of bed without feeling like you want to pass out. Health to you may mean being able to beat your teenage son at 1 on 1 basketball. Health to you may mean getting off all the prescription drugs you are on, or it may mean eating only organic foods and cutting out meat. Fitness, on the other hand, may mean being well rounded in your exercise program, or maybe just taking the dog on a nice walk every evening. Just because you read something or saw a program talking about the value of "Health & Fitness", doesn't mean you will be able to get on board that ship.

The reason it is so important to determine your personal motivation, the exact reason you want to make the change, is because each step in the AOSED process will be tailored specifically to that Awareness.

You may or may not be aware of the study that shows regular physical activity can improve cognitive function and brain health. A recent study conducted at the University of Adelaide in Australia suggests that one thirty minute session of vigorous exercise can lead to changes in the brain that make it more "plastic", including improvements in memory and motor skill coordination.

"Although this was a small sample group, it helps us to better understand the overall picture of how exercise influences the brain," lead researcher Associate Professor Michael Ridding said in a statement. "We know that plasticity is also important for recovery from brain damage, so this opens up potential therapeutic avenues for patients. Further research will be required to see what the possible long-term benefits could be for patients as well as healthy people."

Ridding and his colleagues recruited a small group of adults in their late twenties and early thirties who were asked to ride exercise bikes for a period of thirty minutes. The team of neuroscientists monitored changes in the brain directly after the exercise session and again fifteen minutes later. Results showed that even one thirty-minute session of physical activity can improve the brain's plasticity, or its ability to change physically, functionally and chemically. Positive changes in the brain were sustained fifteen minutes after exercising. "We saw positive changes in the brain straight away and these improvements were sustained 15 minutes after the exercise had ended" Ridding added, "Plasticity in the brain is important for learning, memory and motor skill coordination. The more 'plastic' the brain becomes, the more it's able to reorganize itself, modifying the number and strength of connections between nerve cells and different brain areas. This exercise-related change in the brain may, in part, explain why physical activity has a positive effect on memory and higher-level functions."

That study may do diddly squat for your motivation to exercise for thirty minutes a day because you probably could not care less if your brain has more plasticity. What may be more important to you is the fact that you are sick and tired of being "sick and tired" or, you want to be able to compete in a Spartan obstacle course race and finish just so you can get the free t shirt and wear it to work on Monday. It doesn't matter if your only motivation to work out for thirty minutes is so you can eat 'bonbons' all night and not gain weight. The only thing that matters is...what matters to you. The point here is, if you make it personal, you will have the greatest chance of reaching your desired goal. Your reason never needs to be someone else's reason. We all have different Awareness at different times in our lives. It's the Awareness of the needed change at the present moment which allows us to begin the AOSED process.

Most of us know what we "should be doing" with regard to health and fitness. We have been bombarded with magazines, books, videos, medical research, commercials, programs etc.

that show us all the advantages of being healthy and fit. We admire those who do it and enjoy hearing their success stories. Unfortunately, however, most of us need to hit a wall of some sort before we actually take this seriously, i.e. sickness, near death experience, wakeup call from the doctor, divorce, loss of job, stroke, etc. I am here to show you that, if you are open to it, there is a way you can make a change today. You can choose to go through separate "30 Minute Change" processes, one for health and one for fitness or you can join them together as one single process. It's whatever works best for you.

The next few pages will give you some detailed examples of how to make a change using the Health & Fitness "30 Minute Change" process.

Example 1:

Jamie woke up the other morning, looked in the mirror and became "aware" that the muscle tone he had had in his shoulders for years was gone. He had been very athletic throughout high school and college but for the past few years he has been sitting at a desk all day at work.

That morning, he decided he wanted to change that image in the mirror. He grabbed his "30 Minute Change" summary and strategy sheets, sat down on the couch and started to fill it out.

HEALTH AND FITNESS CHANGE PROCESS FORM

THE AWARENESS: (MUST BE PERSONAL AND DETAILED.)

I have lost the muscle tone in my upper body and shoulders. I will not let myself make any more excuses about it. I need to start working out!

THE OBSTACLE: (MUST BE CLEARLY DETAILED AND DEFINED.)

My work schedule is demanding, I am tired after work and would rather go to eat with my coworkers. It has been a long time since I have worked out.

THE STRATEGY: (MUST BE THOUGHT OUT, DETAILED AND COMMITTED TO.)

I will carve out an hour each lunch break during the week to work out.

WHAT IS THE NEW BELIEF YOU WANT TO HAVE?
(THIS IS A ROUGH DRAFT THOUGHT HERE. YOU WILL CLARIFY LATER IN THE PROCESS.)

I can look like I did in college.

Pros of This Choice	**Cons of This Choice**
I feel great	*Can't go out drinking every night*
I have more energy	*Have to think before I eat*
I drink less beer	
I will get back on a B-Ball team	
My Girlfriend is fired up	
I have more energy at work	
I am driven to compete	
I sleep better	
I eat healthier	
I am back to my desired weight	
Make some new like-minded friends	

(Take your time and write down as many Pros and Cons as you can think of! This helps solidify why this New Belief is valuable to you.)

WHAT THAT NEW STRATEGY LOOKS, SOUNDS AND FEELS LIKE.

Take a moment and close your eyes. Picture yourself already living out this New Belief.

Then describe in detail what you see, hear and feel.

Visual (I see...)

- *I see myself getting out of the car, walking into the gym and saying hello to the trainer.*
- *I see myself in front of the mirror by the dumbbells doing curls and watching my muscles pump up.*
- *I see myself at the beach with the same physique I had four years ago.*

Auditory (I hear...)

- *I hear my coworker's comment about how good I look.*
- *I hear my friend Jeff ask if he can start going to the gym with me at lunch.*
- *I hear the sound of the weights hitting against each other as I lift.*

Kinesthetic (I feel...)

- *I feel energetic. I feel excited to get my work done in the morning so I can take a longer lunch break to work out.*

THE EXECUTION: (MUST BE TIED TO YOUR STRATEGY AND PUT INTO MOTION IMMEDIATELY)

I will talk to my boss this morning and see if I can come to work thirty minutes earlier each day so I can take a longer lunch break to go to the gym. I will stop by the local Gym today after work and renew my membership. I will take out the college picture of me when I was in prime shape and pin it by my desk. I will call my girlfriend and tell her I am joining the gym today.

THE DESIRED RESULT: (THE NEW PERSONAL BELIEF STATEMENT.)

My body is firm, fit and filled with energy from working out every day at lunch.

WHOLE-BRAIN PROGRAMING: (This adds the New Belief to your subconscious. Before starting this final exercise, read though your whole change process form one more time.)

Get into a Whole-Brain Posture (sitting on a chair, legs and arms crossed).

Close your eyes and think about your new desired result belief statement.

"My body is firm, fit and filled with energy from working out every day at lunch."

Concentrate on experiencing a mental, emotional or physical change in your mind and body about your new belief statement as you repeat it over and over again silently.

After a few minutes you will feel a change in your thoughts, feelings or emotions.

Then open your eyes, uncross your body and Lock in the New Belief.

See appendix A in the back of this book for the detailed process of how to do the "Whole-Brain Programing" exercise.

Example 2:

Sherrie is sitting in the doctor's office for the third time this month with high cholesterol and the early stages of kidney failure. Her purse is full of medications prescribed by various doctors and she is beginning to become "aware" that, if she does not make some changes, she may be spending more time in these offices and this honestly make her very afraid.

HEALTH AND FITNESS CHANGE PROCESS FORM

THE AWARENESS: (MUST BE PERSONAL AND DETAILED.)

If I don't change my lifestyle, I may end up in the hospital for months or maybe even dead. I must get some help.

THE OBSTACLE: (MUST BE CLEARLY DETAILED AND DEFINED.)

I love greasy food. I hate exercising. I have way too many TV shows I love to watch. All my friends are afraid to say anything because I get angry at them.

THE STRATEGY: (MUST BE THOUGHT OUT, DETAILED AND COMMITTED TO.)

I will do whatever it takes to lose fifty pounds which means seek input and live to help raise my seven grandchildren.

WHAT IS THE NEW BELIEF YOU WANT TO HAVE? (THIS IS A ROUGH DRAFT THOUGHT HERE. YOU WILL CLARIFY LATER IN THE PROCESS.

I can be healthy and live a long and prosperous life.

Pros of This Choice	Cons of This Choice
I am alive and healthy	*No more excuses*
I look better	*I have to watch what I eat*
I sleep better	*Must break bad habits*
No more fried and greasy food	
I get outside more	
I can garden again	
I am able to spend time with friends	
I get to spend lots of time with family	
I am off all these pills that make me feel terrible	
I am saving money	
I can give away my clothes that are too big	

(Take your time and write down as many Pros and Cons as you can think of! This helps solidify why this New Belief is valuable to you.)

WHAT THAT NEW STRATEGY LOOKS, SOUNDS AND FEELS LIKE.

Take a moment and close your eyes. Picture yourself already living out this New Belief.
Then describe in detail what you see, hear and feel.

Visual (I see...)

- *I see myself standing in the kitchen throwing all my medications in the trash.*
- *I see myself going to the store and shopping for a whole new size twelve wardrobe.*

- *I see myself picking up my grandchildren and kissing them over and over again.*

Auditory (I hear...)

- *I hear my granddaughter Madison telling me, "You look so healthy Ma Ma".*
- *I hear my doctor tell me he can't believe the speed at which I made the changes.*
- *I hear my neighbor William asking me, "What did you do to look so healthy?"*

Kinesthetic (I feel...)

- *I feel healthy. I feel excited to wake up and get out of bed to walk one mile every morning. I feel like I have the energy I did when I was thirty.*

THE EXECUTION: (MUST BE TIED TO YOUR STRATEGY AND PUT INTO MOTION IMMEDIATELY.)

I will sit down and watch the documentary "Fat, Sick and Nearly Dead" that my brother has been wanting me to watch. I will agree with my neighbor Claudia to go walking between twenty and thirty minutes every day. I will tell my doctor today that I will go to the diet class he has been pushing me to go to for years. I will only watch two hours of TV a day.

THE DESIRED RESULT: (THE NEW PERSONAL BELIEF STATEMENT.)

I am light, healthy and medication free!

WHOLE-BRAIN PROGRAMING: (This adds the New Belief to your subconscious. Before starting this final exercise, read though your whole change process form one more time.)

Get into a Whole-Brain Posture (sitting on a chair, legs and arms crossed).
Close your eyes and think about your new desired result belief statement.

"I am light, healthy and medication free!"

Concentrate on experiencing a mental, emotional or physical change in your mind and body about your new belief statement

as you repeat it over and over again silently.

After a few minutes you will feel a change in your thoughts, feelings or emotions.

Then open your eyes, uncross your body and Lock in the New Belief.

Example 3:

Steve just became *aware* he may be addicted to caffeine and sugar. After tossing and turn all night, as usual, he woke up and began to think about his daily routine. He starts his day with a double espresso and a sugary muffin. When he gets to the office, he has an energy drink to keep the work flowing. For lunch, he usually goes out and almost always has a soda or two. In the afternoon he has another energy drink and/or a candy bar. Dinner is light with dessert and a few beers. Steve is ready to make a change. What is so crazy to him is that he knows better. He has read "The 30 Minute Change" and even used the process and work sheets to find the killer job he is in now. Steve pulls out the Health work sheets and sits at the table.

HEALTH AND FITNESS CHANGE PROCESS FORM

THE AWARENESS: (MUST BE PERSONAL AND DETAILED.)

I am totally addicted to caffeine and sugar. I love the highs but the lows have just surpassed the highs and I am done!

THE OBSTACLE: (MUST BE CLEARLY DETAILED AND DEFINED.)

This is something I have been doing for years. What will give me the energy I need? Can I find a substitute to pick me up?

THE STRATEGY: (MUST BE THOUGHT OUT, DETAILED AND COMMITTED TO.)

I will avoid all opportunities to consume caffeine and sugar. Take yoga or some form of meditation class to help slow me down.

WHAT IS THE NEW BELIEF YOU WANT TO HAVE?
(THIS IS A ROUGH DRAFT THOUGHT HERE. YOU WILL CLARIFY LATER IN THE PROCESS.)

I control my mood swings

Pros of This Choice	**Cons of This Choice**
No more mood swings	*Can't eat anything I want*
Have steadier energy levels	*Will feel worse before better*
Start working out again	*My friends will razz me.*
Find more peace	
Gain healthy weight	
My girlfriend will be happier	
I will feel healthier	
Will be able to control my eating	
Open to new adventures	

(Take your time and write down as many Pros and Cons as you can think of! This helps solidify why this New Belief is valuable to you.)

WHAT THAT NEW STRATEGY LOOKS, SOUNDS AND FEELS LIKE.

Take a moment and close your eyes. Picture yourself already living out this New Belief.
Then describe in detail what you see, hear and feel.

Visual (I see...)

- *I see myself gaining fifteen pounds and getting back to my former weight in high school.*
- *I see myself walking right by the vending machine with a no-sugar protein bar in my hand.*
- *I see myself sitting calmly in the park reading a book and enjoying the sun on my face.*

Auditory (I hear...)

- *I hear my coworkers talking about how calm I seem.*
- *I hear the birds sing as I jog past the large oak tree at Kettering Park*
- *I hear my dad saying how proud he is of the changes I have made.*

Kinesthetic (I feel...)

- *I feel completely peaceful and happy, I feel totally in tune with my surroundings. I feel in control.*

THE EXECUTION: (MUST BE TIED TO YOUR STRATEGY AND PUT INTO MOTION IMMEDIATELY.)

I will have one cup of coffee in the morning with no sugar, I will use Stevia. I will cut out candy, soda and energy drinks at work and substitute them with healthy choices. When I have the feeling that I need a pick me up, I will go outside and take a "slow walk" and concentrate on my breathing. I will not stop at 7-Eleven on the way to work. I will go and take three yoga classes a week with my girlfriend.

THE DESIRED RESULT: (THE NEW PERSONAL BELIEF STATEMENT.)

I eat and drink only things that bring me peace and health!

WHOLE-BRAIN PROGRAMING: (This adds the New Belief to your subconscious. Before starting this final exercise, read though your whole change process form one more time.)

Get into a Whole-Brain Posture (sitting on a chair, legs and arms crossed).
Close your eyes and think about your new desired result belief statement.

"I eat and drink only things that bring me peace and health."

Concentrate on experiencing a mental, emotional or physical change in your mind and body about your new belief statement as you repeat it over and over again silently.
After a few minutes you will feel a change in your thoughts, feelings or emotions.
Then open your eyes, uncross your body and Lock in the New Belief.

Other possible example of Awareness with regard to Health & Fitness:

- I want to go work out five days a week.
- I need to re-watch "Fat, Sick and Nearly Dead"
- I need to join a hiking meet up.
- I will find someone to go with to an AAA meeting.
- I will stop smoking marijuana.
- I want to run a half marathon.
- I need to stop eating after seven p.m.
- I want to take thirty minutes a day to mediate and pray.
- I will walk to work Mon, Wed & Fri.
- Etc....

Bonus: If you feel you would like to get some help just getting started on any of the change processes, we have a one on one personal coaching session available for you. It is a focused 90-minute training session done over the phone. This will help walk you through one or two needed changes in detail, the only goal being, that when you are done with that one session, you will be equipped to take yourself-through any of your needed changes in 30 minutes or less. This is a great option for some and has had tremendous success.

Visit: www.30MinuteChange.com to find out more.

Chapter 6

Finances

"It doesn't matter how many times you fall down
As long as you have the means to pay someone to pick you up."

This has got to be one of the biggest areas in which most of us have had the least amount of training. In my High School in the 80s (and from what I have seen with my four kids it hasn't changed much), we spent three years learning how to properly write a term paper, being taught about the history of cultures most of us would never see or think about again, plus three years studying higher levels of mathematics for which we can now find the solutions, one hundred times faster, on our phones. However, with teaching about the basics of budgets, debt to income ratios, assets versus liabilities, compounded interest, managing debt or the great advantage of the "one-day rule", there's been no progress. For those of you wondering what the "one-day rule" is, it is the system of protecting yourself from buying on an impulse. Take twenty-four hours and then see if you still want and need it.

For me personally, this is an area I have lived most of my life walking aimlessly around in. My father was a successful vice president at one of the largest breweries in the world. He was able to retire at forty-five and move to the country to live out his passion of fixing up old Cadillacs. He was very wise with his money and was a CPA. I never in my life saw him use a credit card. He never paid anyone to fix anything around our house. We never moved or bought anything new. He always gave something to the church or the poor. But... he never taught me a thing about money. We never discussed the value of money or the problems it can create. I remember asking him how much money he made and he quickly avoided the subject. We never discussed budgets, assets versus liabilities, compounded interest, managing debt or anything along those lines. I was left believing that if you work hard, you can always have money. So, I always worked to have money but never thought about having my money work hard for me. I also believed that any success I had financially in my life would also include a lot of luck or being in the right place at the right time.

What I have now learned, is that those who have been educated or continue to seek more education with regard to the many facets of finances, seem to always maintain a steady life flow. Not a lot of ups and not a lot of downs. I remember reading books like, "The Millionaire Next Door". and, "Rich Dad Poor Dad", and feeling like I was only in preschool when it came to my knowledge of money. That is where my understanding of the value of seeking advice and learning from those more knowledgeable than myself took root. Since my early thirties, I have continued to educate myself in many different areas of the financial world. My biggest problem was not learning the information, believe me I have that down, my problem has always been actually implementing that knowledge. There were times when I thought I would also retire by the age of forty-five and then a few years later I was flat broke and having to completely start over, always telling myself, "If I only knew then, what I know now."

To have true financial success, there must come a point in all of our lives where we need to start "knowing now, so we don't have to find out then." The two biggest factors, in my opinion, that play the largest role in any financial plan must be humility, and willingness to seek advice. Why pretend any longer that you have this part of your life down? Who are you really trying to fool? Why not make today the day you change your misguided or misinformed views about your finances... and I'll start!

This was the chapter I was putting off until the end, because it is one of my biggest weaknesses. This subject is something I avoid talking about, thinking about or wanting to deal with, due to my many past mistakes and beliefs. Remember: "Everything I have seen, heard and felt in my past determines how I see, hear and feel things today." So as to not be a total hypocrite, I myself will be going through the "30 Minute Change" process as one of the three examples below, (I will save mine until the end.)

Example 1:

Jeremey has no savings account. He doesn't mind working hard and has a job that pays well. He has had three promotions in the last seven years. He is thirty-two years old and still single. He drives a brand-new Ford Mustang GT, rents a nice one bedroom in the city and likes to travel three to four times a year. One night, Jeremey woke from a dream where he was homeless, living on the streets and was begging for money from his best friend Tyron.

That next morning, he sat at the kitchen table, took out a piece of paper and wrote out his budget and then his debt to income ratio. He quickly became aware that he was only one lay off or firing away from having to sell most of his stuff to keep his condo for the next month until he could find another job. This was motivation enough for him to start the detailed Financial change process form.

FINANCIAL CHANGE PROCESS FORM

THE AWARENESS: (MUST BE PERSONAL AND DETAILED.)
I have no savings and my spending has "no control."

THE OBSTACLE: (MUST BE CLEARLY DETAILED AND DEFINED.)
I love to eat what I want, buy what I want and do what I want. I do not follow a budget. I have a habit of living financially day to day.

THE STRATEGY: (MUST BE THOUGHT OUT, DETAILED AND COMMITTED TO.)
Get on a budget! Pay off debt. Plan for the future.

WHAT IS THE NEW BELIEF YOU WANT TO HAVE?
(THIS IS A ROUGH DRAFT THOUGHT HERE. YOU WILL CLARIFY LATER IN THE PROCESS.)

I am disciplined and wise with my money.

Pros of This Choice	**Cons of This Choice**
I will be out of debt	*Have to be disciplined*
I will be less stressed	*Can't buy whatever I want*

118

Pros of This Choice	Cons of This Choice
I can travel more	*Have to be on a budget*
I can sell stuff I don't need	
I can save to buy a place of my own	
I will have savings	
I can help those in need	
I will feel better about myself	
I will sleep better	
I can find a wife	
I will retire younger	

(Take your time and write down as many Pros and Cons as you can think of! This helps solidify why this New Belief is valuable to you.)

WHAT THAT NEW STRATEGY LOOKS, SOUNDS AND FEELS LIKE.

Take a moment and close your eyes. Picture yourself already living out this New Belief.
Then describe in detail what you see, hear and feel.

Visual (I see...)

- *I see myself opening my bank statement showing $25,000 in savings.*
- *I see myself walking out of the electronics store without buying anything.*
- *I see myself sign escrow papers on my new townhome.*

Auditory (I hear...)

- *I hear my mom thanking me for taking her on vacation.*
- *I hear my buddy Tyron saying, "man you're really on top of things."*
- *I hear the music playing as I sit on the deck at my new place.*

Kinesthetic (I feel...)

- *I feel in control. I feel peaceful. I feel smart.*

THE EXECUTION: (MUST BE TIED TO YOUR STRATEGY AND PUT INTO MOTION IMMEDIATELY)

Tonight, after work, solidify my budget in writing. Sign up for a Dave Ramsey class online. Call Michelle and ask her to start showing me townhomes so I can get a vision of what I need to do.

THE DESIRED RESULT: (YOUR NEW PERSONAL BELIEF STATEMENT.)

I work successfully with my finances and they work with me.

WHOLE-BRAIN PROGRAMING: (This adds the New Belief to your subconscious. Before starting this final exercise, read though your whole change process form one more time.)

Get into a Whole-Brain Posture (sitting on a chair, legs and arms crossed).
Close your eyes and think about your new desired result belief statement.

"I work successfully with my finances and they work with me."

Concentrate on experiencing a mental, emotional or physical change in your mind and body about your New Belief statement as you repeat it over and over again silently.
After a few minutes you will feel a change in your thoughts, feeling or emotions.
Then open your eyes, uncross your body and Lock in the New Belief.

See appendix A in the back of this book for the detailed process of how to do the "Whole-Brain Programing" exercise.

Example 2:

Tammy is a business owner who has owned and operated her own yogurt shop for over eight years. She has been talking about expanding the business for the last three years but seems to keep finding excuses. She knows she will never be able to help pay for her kids' college with the proceeds of this one shop. After going to a women's small business seminar, Tammy

120

finally faces her fears and becomes aware that she does not know where to start the process for expanding her business.

FINANCIAL CHANGE PROCESS FORM

THE AWARENESS: (MUST BE PERSONAL AND DETAILED.)

I need to open another yogurt shop.

THE OBSTACLE: (MUST BE CLEARLY DETAILED AND DEFINED.)

Do not know where to start. I am afraid of failure. Don't have the money. Have no help and work too much as it is.

THE STRATEGY: (MUST BE THOUGHT OUT, DETAILED AND COMMITTED TO.)

Join the local chamber and meet other small business owners. Set up a meeting with my accountant to see if he has any ideas. Meet with my banker about a business loan. Raise up a new manager.

WHAT IS THE NEW BELIEF YOU WANT TO HAVE?
(THIS IS A ROUGH DRAFT THOUGHT HERE. YOU WILL CLARIFY LATER IN THE PROCESS.)

I can open my second location this year.

Pros of This Choice	Cons of This Choice
I will own two stores	*Can't procrastinate anymore*
I will make more money	*Taking a financial risk*
I can hire my friends' kids	*More challenges ahead*
I will increase my faith	
I will be able to pay for college	
I can retire sooner	
I may franchise one day	
I will feel better about myself	
I will learn a lot from others	
I will conquer my fears	
I will make new friends	
I will be very successful	

(Take your time and write down as many Pros and Cons as you can think of! This helps solidify why this New Belief is valuable to you.)

WHAT THAT NEW STRATEGY LOOKS, SOUNDS AND FEELS LIKE.

Take a moment and close your eyes. Picture yourself already living out this New Belief.
Then describe in detail what you see, hear and feel.

Visual (I see...)

- *I see myself signing the loan papers at the bank.*
- *I see the sign going up at my new location.*
- *I see myself mingling with other business owners and exchanging business cards.*

Auditory (I hear...)

- *I hear my daughter tell me how proud she is of me taking this risk.*
- *I hear my customers telling me they love the new location.*
- *I hear my accountant tell me we doubled the profit this year.*

Kinesthetic (I feel...)

- *I feel empowered. I feel confident. I feel joyful.*

THE EXECUTION: (MUST BE TIED TO YOUR STRATEGY AND PUT INTO MOTION IMMEDIATELY)

Call my accountant and banker today to set up a meeting for this week. Join the chamber today. Read a book on how to grow my business. Raise up Trisha to be the manager so I can focus on this new endeavor.

THE DESIRED RESULT: (YOUR NEW PERSONAL BELIEF STATEMENT.)
I am a successful business owner of two incredibly popular yogurt shops.

WHOLE-BRAIN PROGRAMING: (This adds the New Belief to your subconscious. Before starting this final exercise, read though your whole change process form one more time.)

Get into a Whole-Brain Posture (sitting on a chair, legs and arms crossed). Close your eyes and think about your new desired result belief statement.

"I am a successful business owner of two incredible yogurt shops."

Concentrate on experiencing a mental, emotional or physical change in your mind and body about your New Belief statement as you repeat it over and over again silently.
After a few minutes you will feel a change in your thoughts, feeling or emotions.
Then open your eyes, uncross your body and Lock in the New Belief.

Example 3:

Finally, it's my turn! Time to face my needed change of being consistently involved in our finances.

FINANCIAL CHANGE PROCESS FORM

THE AWARENESS: (MUST BE PERSONAL AND DETAILED.)

I avoid looking at my finances. I leave it all to my wife who is not happy I am not engaged. I just want to keep working hard, taking risks and getting by.

THE OBSTACLE: (MUST BE CLEARLY DETAILED AND DEFINED.)

I am a conflict avoider. I like to wing it. I lack self-discipline. I like to be in control.

THE STRATEGY: (MUST BE THOUGHT OUT, DETAILED AND COMMITTED TO.)

Work together with my wife. Develop short term and long-term goals. Execute a savings plan and stick to it.

WHAT IS THE NEW BELIEF YOU WANT TO HAVE?
(THIS IS A ROUGH DRAFT THOUGHT HERE. YOU WILL CLARIFY LATER IN THE PROCESS.)

I love dealing with my personal finances.

123

Pros of This Choice	**Cons of This Choice**
My wife will be thrilled	*Can't do anything I want*
I will be more self-controlled	*Face my fears*
I will gain more wisdom	*Deal with conflict*
I can plan my future	
Give more money away	
Train my kids through my mistakes	
Be less stressed	
Lead by example for my readers	
Take more vacations	
Live abroad a few months a year	
Won't have that feeling in my stomach	
Be more focused and attentive	

(Take your time and write down as many Pros and Cons as you can think of! This helps solidify why this New Belief is valuable to you.)

WHAT THAT NEW STRATEGY LOOKS, SOUNDS AND FEELS LIKE.

Take a moment and close your eyes. Picture yourself already living out this New Belief.
Then describe in detail what you see, hear and feel.

Visual (I see...)

- *I see myself sitting with my wife at the kitchen table every week talking through our finances and budget.*
- *I see myself teaching a class one day on this subject.*
- *I see myself able to give to anyone in need without needing to be paid back.*

Auditory (I hear...)

- *I hear my wife thanking me for getting involved & keeping my head out of the sand.*
- *I hear people asking me for financial advice.*
- *I hear my pastor asking me to teach a class on self-discipline.*

Kinesthetic (I feel...)

- *I feel empowered. I feel at peace. I feel engaged.*

THE EXECUTION: (MUST BE TIED TO YOUR STRATEGY AND PUT INTO MOTION IMMEDIATELY)

Tonight, I will apologize to my wife for my lack of effort in becoming more involved in our finances and set a time each week to review. Come up with an agreed savings plan and start it right away. Seek more advice from my friend Dominic who is great at this.

THE DESIRED RESULT: (YOUR NEW PERSONAL BELIEF STATEMENT.)

I happily control and grow my finances together with my wife.

WHOLE-BRAIN PROGRAMING: (This adds the New Belief to your subconscious. Before starting this final exercise, read though your whole change process form one more time.)

Get into a Whole-Brain Posture (sitting on a chair, legs and arms crossed).
Close your eyes and think about your new desired result belief statement.

"I happily control and grow my finances together with my wife."

Concentrate on experiencing a mental, emotional or physical change in your mind and body about your New Belief statement as you repeat it over and over again silently.
After a few minutes you will feel a change in your thoughts, feeling or emotions.
Then open your eyes, uncross your body and Lock in the New Belief.

That was good! I feel much better now and focused on what I need to do to make this change. For me, this was a good chapter to work through. I had been avoiding writing it for weeks, thinking I had nothing to share here. Doing this exercise, myself never even crossed my mind, which is odd since I am writing a book on this process, coach many through it and know how well it works. But again, it just proves the fact that until you have personal awareness that you really want and need to make a change in your life, it won't happen. It will only remain a random thought you have when you're feeling emotional about it.

Other possible examples of Awareness in regard to Financial change:

- I need to make a will or living trust.
- I don't make enough money at my current job.
- I need to teach my kids some of the basics I was never taught.
- I need to lower my debt.
- I need to start tithing 10%.
- I need to buy an income property.
- I need to hire a Fiduciary money manager.
- I need to downsize our house.
- I would like to teach a free class on money managing to single moms.
- I want to start investing 10% of everything I make.
- Etc.

The changes you will make by taking the time to go through one of these exercises will amaze you. You can take out a piece of paper and do this anytime you want to make a change or, if you would like to download a set of "Change Process" forms that are already created for you to just fill in, they are available for download at: **www.30MinuteChange.com**

Chapter 7

Weight Control

*"Remember...It's not where you look, it's what you see.
So you don't have to move to get a better view,
Just change what you see."*

I am not calling this chapter, 'Weight Loss', because that term has caused more tension in the lives of wonderful people than any of us can even imagine. We all know that we can lose weight, but the real problem is that the weight seems to find its way back, and quickly. I would like to introduce the term "Weight Control" into your belief system instead, with the fact that, when we can gain control of our weight, we will become empowered to maintain that control. For many of us, the problem is that we are not consistent and thus never actually gain control, but rather we keep bouncing from one diet fad to the next, one program to the next, this class or that class, this book or that book, we take out foods from our diet or put new ones in, take new supplements or diet pills and, truthfully, this just shows how "out of control" we really are. Therefore, I am suggesting that we take control of our weight and feel the power that comes along with this New Belief. This chapter will help you learn how to make the necessary belief changes to gain control of your weight.

Really, what is weight loss? What does it mean to lose

weight? What is the description of weight and who defined weight in your life and what does that mean to you? Weight is a clearly distinct subject, but weight loss is relative. Why don't you substitute the idea of losing weight with something that is very constructive, positive, encouraging and attainable? For example, seeing, feeling, and executing weight control in your life is very empowering. Webster's defines "control" as "to exercise constraint or direct influence over something, to have power over, to reduce the severity of." You can gain control over your weight. It's as easy as creating a New Belief about that fact.

Let's talk about how you can gain "Weight Control" by becoming more aware of the fact that you already have the proper control within you.

How do you know if you do not have control of your weight? Rather than list one hundred different ways here, I will sum it up in one: if you are not perfectly happy with your current weight, then you are <u>not</u> in control. Please understand that there are many outside influences that may be causing you to be unhappy with your weight. For example:

- There's something in my life that's making me very unhappy and I'm eating to ease the pain
- My significant other keeps telling me to lose weight
- I need to look like the people on TV or in the magazines
- My mom has always said I am fat
- Food is my only pleasure
- My significant other eats a lot so I feel I have to as well
- Eating helps me escape

- I am addicted to sugar
- Etc....

The Weight Control change process will only work if you take the time to clearly define what is causing you the unhappiness with your weight. If you believe it goes deeper, which in most every case it does, I suggest you spend time first in the "Personal Growth" chapter of this book and work through a few changes there before you tackle "Weight Control".

Additionally, if your unhappiness only stems from other people's Awareness of your weight, that will not be enough to make the change; it must come from a "personal awareness" that you are not in control and want to be. If you are perfectly happy with your weight and it's just everyone else that has a problem with it, then you have nothing to change here, they do!

All that being said, however, I have found that most people fall into the category of personal discontentment with their weight. Therefore, we will go through a few examples of the "Weight Control" AOSED change process now.

Example: What's the awareness? I'm overweight!

Sometimes a vague awareness is not as helpful, so let's be more specific here and let's say you're fifty plus pounds overweight. You didn't start out that overweight, you slowly gained a pound a week for the past year and now all of a sudden, you realize you are fifty-two pounds overweight. You didn't notice at first because you saw yourself every day and the progression was so slow that it was hard to see. Even those around you may not have noticed right away because they too may have been slowly gaining weight, (I do not mean to be critical or judgmental here, but have you ever been in an office environment where the majority of the staff is noticeably overweight and so no one is really aware of each other's weight gain, let alone their own). Maybe your spouse does notice and wants you to lose fifty pounds, but that's his/her awareness, not yours. Until your need for weight control becomes your own awareness, there is no point in implementing the next three steps because they will not produce the results intended.

But, let's assume you have become aware of the situation. *This is good!*

Step one: What's the Awareness?

Now your answer will change, from, "I'm overweight", to, "I am fifty-two pounds over my desired weight and want to do something about it NOW!"
Okay, what's the Obstacle?

Is it: I love eating? I drink too much beer? I eat way too much at night before bed? I eat until I'm stuffed? Honestly, I don't even realize I'm eating so much? There's something in my life that's making me very unhappy and I'm eating to ease the pain, (again, if that is the case, stop here and go to the "Personal Growth" 30-minute change process first) etc.

What's the Strategy? As it will be different for each one of these statements, let's start with the Obstacle: *"I eat until I'm stuffed"*

I will focus my attention on eating smaller portions, fifty percent of what I'm currently eating at each meal and add a small, healthy snack between meals.

The Execution? *This will depend on your specific situation but here are some* options:

Let your wife know you want half portions from now on. When you go out to restaurants, set up a plan to share a meal with somebody or ask your server for a smaller size. Every day, bring two small sized snacks with you: apples and almonds, a banana or yogurt, a piece of fruit and a no sugar protein bar. Find a picture of yourself when you weighed the weight that you want to be now and hang it on the bathroom mirror, put it in your car, stick it in your cubicle or shrink it and put it by your wallet. Whatever it takes!

Here's the deal. If you don't break it down like this with a very clear definition of your Obstacles, followed by a very clear definition of your Strategies and a very detailed Execution, you will not reach your Desired Result, which is your wanted New Belief about this change.

But what's so cool is that, on the flipside, if you define your Obstacle, define your Strategy, define and implement your Execution, you will receive the Desired Result!

Okay, now let's look at some detailed examples and apply them to the "Weight Control" change forms:

Example 1:

Roger is a single dad who works hard and has many

friends. He has noticed for years how his weight goes up and down three or four times a year. Each year it has been going up more and not coming down as far. He is finally ready to do something about it.

WEIGHT CONTROL CHANGE PROCESS FORM

THE AWARENESS: (MUST BE PERSONAL AND DETAILED.)

My weight fluctuates ten to twenty pounds every few months. I need to control my eating habits.

THE OBSTACLE: (MUST BE CLEARLY DETAILED AND DEFINED.)

I eat healthily for a week or so and then slip back into old habits. I am very undisciplined in my eating choices. I eat even when I am not hungry.

THE STRATEGY: (MUST BE THOUGHT OUT, DETAILED AND COMMITTED TO.)

I need to define what I should eat and what I should not eat. I need to find other things to do other than eat when I am bored. I need an accountability partner.

WHAT IS THE NEW BELIEF YOU WANT TO HAVE?
(THIS IS A ROUGH DRAFT THOUGHT HERE. YOU WILL CLARIFY LATER IN THE PROCESS.)

I have control over what I eat and need help making good food decisions.

Pros of This Choice:	Cons of This Choice:
I will look good	*Can't eat anything I want*
I will gain control	*Can't eat anytime I want*
I will find new things to do	*Must plan my meals*
I can get rid of my second set of clothes	
I will be motivated to exercise	
I will gain discipline	
My kids will be happy for me	
I will feel better about myself	
I will sleep better	

Pros of This Choice:	Cons of This Choice:
My doctor will be impressed *I will be in better health* *I will only eat what makes me feel good* *I can get off some of my medications*	

(Take your time and write down as many Pros and Cons as you can think of! This helps solidify why this New Belief is valuable to you.)

WHAT THAT NEW STRATEGY LOOKS, SOUNDS AND FEELS LIKE.

Take a moment and close your eyes. Picture yourself already living out this New Belief.
Then describe in detail what you see, hear and feel.

Visual (I see...)

- *I see myself driving my "Big" clothes to the Salvation Army.*
- *I see myself sitting in my favorite restaurant ordering healthy choices and smiling.*
- *I see my son and I taking long walks together because I can breathe easier.*

Auditory (I hear...)

- *I hear my daughter whisper in my ear that she thinks I look great.*
- *I hear my neighbor Alex asking me. "what's different about you?"*
- *I hear my pastor asking me to teach a class on self-discipline.*

Kinesthetic (I feel...)

- *I feel healthy. I feel energetic and light. I feel happy.*

THE EXECUTION: (MUST BE TIED TO YOUR STRATEGY AND PUT INTO MOTION IMMEDIATELY.)

Tonight, I will throw away all the stuff I know I shouldn't be eating.

I will sit down and write a defined meal plan tomorrow. After that I will invite Ari over and ask him to help keep me accountable. He is a health freak. When I am bored, I will get up and take a short walk to encourage my New Belief.

THE DESIRED RESULT: (YOUR NEW PERSONAL BELIEF STATEMENT.)

I am in total control of my body and what I choose to put in it.

WHOLE-BRAIN PROGRAMING: (This adds the New Belief to your subconscious. Before starting this final exercise, read though your whole change process form one more time.)

Get into a Whole-Brain Posture (sitting on a chair, legs and arms crossed).
Close your eyes and think about your new desired result belief statement.

"I am in total control of my body and what I choose to put in it."

Concentrate on experiencing a mental, emotional or physical change in your mind and body about your New Belief statement as you repeat it over and over again silently.
After a few minutes you will feel a change in your thoughts, feelings or emotions.
Then open your eyes, uncross your body and Lock in the New Belief.

See appendix A in the back of this book for the detailed process of how to do the "Whole-Brain Programing" exercise.

Example 2:

Nicole is a successful businesswoman living in a major metropolitan city. She has been hearing for years how "thin" she is getting. It has always gone in one ear and out the other. Before, she thought it was just her family and friends being their usual critical selves but now she is actually concerned for her wellbeing.

WEIGHT CONTROL CHANGE PROCESS FORM

THE AWARENESS: (MUST BE PERSONAL AND DETAILED.)

I am too skinny. My clothes fall off of me. I look sickly most of the time. I am not happy with the way I look. I am always on the go and forget to eat.

THE OBSTACLE: (MUST BE CLEARLY DETAILED AND DEFINED.)

If I am not hungry, I don't eat. I know smoking curbs my appetite. I think I am addicted to caffeine and sugar. I don't like to shop for food.

THE STRATEGY: (MUST BE THOUGHT OUT, DETAILED AND COMMITTED TO.)

Eat more often. Cut down on caffeine and sugar. Try to quit smoking. Eat more protein. Keep food in my fridge.

WHAT IS THE NEW BELIEF YOU WANT TO HAVE?
(THIS IS A ROUGH DRAFT THOUGHT HERE. YOU WILL CLARIFY LATER IN THE PROCESS.)

I am healthy and look like I used to when I ate well and took care of myself.

Pros of This Choice	**Cons of This Choice**
I have natural energy	*I am used to living this way*
I look great in a dress	*Can't make any more excuses*
My mom will be thrilled	*I will have to quit smoking*
I will be more attractive to men	*I love sugar and caffeine*
I gain power and trust in myself	
I look in the mirror and feel good	
I won't be so depressed	
No more sugar blues	
I will have more opportunities at work	
People will stop making comments	

Pros of This Choice	Cons of This Choice
I can get a new wardrobe	
Find more peace and joy	

(Take your time and write down as many Pros and Cons as you can think of! This helps solidify why this New Belief is valuable to you.)

WHAT THAT NEW STRATEGY LOOKS, SOUNDS AND FEELS LIKE.

Take a moment and close your eyes. Picture yourself already living out this New Belief.
Then describe in detail what you see, hear and feel.

Visual (I see...)

I see myself filled out and my face is healthy and full.

I see my mother walk in the door and her face in total shock at how good I look.

I see myself at the club with my friends and I am the only one not smoking.

Auditory (I hear...)

- *I hear my boss telling me how healthy I look.*
- *I hear my friends talking about all the changes I have made.*
- *I hear my mom tell me how proud she is of me.*

Kinesthetic (I feel...)

- *I feel fantastic. I feel powerful. I feel like I can do anything I want. I feel content with myself.*

THE EXECUTION: (MUST BE TIED TO YOUR STRATEGY AND PUT INTO MOTION IMMEDIATELY.)

I will cut down my smoking to two a day. I will not have coffee until I have had breakfast. I will limit my coffee to one cup a day. I will cut out energy drinks altogether. I will ask Desiree to go grocery shopping with me. I will gain fifteen pounds in the next two months by seeking advice and reading books on healthy weight gain.

THE DESIRED RESULT: (YOUR NEW PERSONAL BELIEF STATEMENT.)

I understand the value of my health and make wise choices every day!

WHOLE-BRAIN PROGRAMING: (This adds the New Belief to your subconscious. Before starting this final exercise, read though your whole change process form one more time.)

Get into a Whole-Brain Posture (sitting on a chair, legs and arms crossed).
Close your eyes and think about your new desired result belief statement.

"I understand the value of my health and make wise choices every day!"

Concentrate on experiencing a mental, emotional or physical change in your mind and body about your New Belief statement as you repeat it over and over again silently.
After a few minutes you will feel a change in your thoughts, feelings or emotions.
Then open your eyes, uncross your body and Lock in the New Belief.

Final thoughts on this subject.

As you can probably tell, I am not a health and nutrition expert. I have read many books and take great care of myself because I believe that to have a healthy mind, you have a much better chance with a healthy body. The advice I give you in this chapter is only to help you become aware of the value of being in control of your weight and defining what that means to you. I also believe this is an area where many will need an accountability partner, someone to encourage, challenge and inspire the Desired Change. This is something I suggest you add to your Strategy and Execution.

Other possible examples of Awareness with regard to Weight Control:

- I eat way too many carbs.
- I eat only one real meal a day.
- I know the good I ought to do but don't do it.
- I need to cut out bread completely.
- I do not eat enough protein.
- I need to try being gluten free for thirty days and see what happens.
- I felt much better when I was vegetarian. I need to do that again.
- When I cut bread and sugar out of my diet I lost twenty pounds. I will do that now.
- I need to enroll back with Weight Watchers.
- I need to find a weight control partner.
- Etc.

The changes you will make by taking the time to go through one of these exercises will amaze you. You can take out a piece of paper and do this anytime you want to make a change or, if you would like to download a set of "Change Process" forms that are already created for you to just fill in, they are available for download at: **www.30MinuteChange.com**

Chapter 8

Parenting

"There is no greater challenge than looking into your own eyes.
Until your own eyes grow up and look back at you."

I have been humbled many times in my life through various situations but I never understood the meaning of the word until I started raising teenagers. I understand now why my parents never cared much if I was home. I thought they were giving me freedom but really, it was freedom for them.

How many times have we heard it said, "If I only knew then, what I know now?" Well that can be a true statement for just about everything in our lives. Not that it means much and is not very helpful or encouraging in the moment, that is unless it brings an Awareness to the fact that you can learn 'now', what you needed to know then.

Being a parent is for life. There is no other occupation in the world about which you can say that. You may be a student, laborer, pro athlete, sculptor, banker, actor, spouse, world leader, criminal, judge, etc....for a short time, but you are a parent, literally, until death do you part. So that being said, this is something you are going to want to get right, no matter how long it takes. In my opinion and experience from many years of counselling and mentoring many different types of people, the common thread through eighty percent plus, is past issues with a parent. Why is that? Everyone has their own theories on that question. To me, it comes down to the fact that most parents have absolutely no idea what they are doing. They just subconsciously transfer everything they have seen, heard or felt in their own past onto the lives of their children. And most of what they have seen, heard and felt was passed down from previous generations to the next, not the genes, but the beliefs and actions based on those beliefs. Why do you think racism and hatred for other cultures are still just as strong today as they were hundreds or even thousands of years ago? Why is there generation after generation of families still on welfare? Why is child abuse today worse than it was one hundred years ago? I say because it is being passed on through the beliefs, which determine the actions, from one to another.

Examples: When you're a single parent and had a bad break up with your spouse and now you find yourself talking bad about all members of the opposite sex to justify your hurt and anger; when you talk down a certain group or a race of people; when you are afraid of everything around you; when you attack first and ask questions later; when you feel better putting others down; when you are a blame shifter and can never take responsibility etc. All of these and hundreds more will have a direct effect on your children, just as they have had on you. You say, "I do it behind their backs, or when they are asleep". Don't kid yourself. Children are super intelligent and aware and feed off your energy. Remember, out of the mouth overflows the heart.

The great news is, once you become aware that you are in fact, NOT a product of your past, and just because your parents/grandparents did or didn't do this or that, doesn't mean you are destined to do the same, thankfully, you will realize that you live in times where you have more freedom to make choices and changes than your predecessors had. The only question is therefore, will you? Will you make the effort to change and create "New Beliefs" about your present and future? Will you allow yourself the freedom to let go of your faulty subconscious programs? Will you take back the power that comes from taking the time to implement the AOSED change process? And, so far as this chapter goes, will you set the example and teach your children to do the same?

I do not have time in this book to go into all the details that will help you understand that we are all just blank tapes from the time we are born until about the age of six or seven, subconsciously recording everything we see and hear, (I suggest you read "The Biology of Belief" by Bruce Lipton which goes into greater detail). This means, as parents with this new Awareness, we now understand that we have tremendous control over how our children view not only themselves, but the people around them and everything else in the world. That is a lot of power in the hands of a parent! The sad thing is, many of those parents have no right wielding that kind of power; their backgrounds and the experiences of what they have seen, heard and felt will directly affect how they parent. I know this is something they probably told themselves before they had children - "I will be different, I will never do that to my kids." Great intentions no doubt! But, over time, they find themselves uncontrollably slipping into the subconscious programs that are controlling them and, before they know it, someone says, "You're just like your father" or, "You're just like your mother." And they're like, "NO, DON'T SAY THAT!"

May I suggest that many of you fall into the above example to one degree or another. How could it be otherwise? There are eight thousand seven hundred and sixty hours in a year. Let's just say you spend fifty percent of the first seven years with your parents (that's minus sleep and some school). That is over sixty-one thousand hours of programming into your hungry brain. What other entity out there has had that much influence over you? In many cases, that programming your parents gave you was faulty but what did you know? Your brain did not yet have the cognitive ability to decipher the truth. It just believed what it was told. So, going forward, for you as a parent, how valuable would it be for you to start reprogramming some faulty recordings in your subconscious? Would your children not benefit from that? It's never too late to start.

Here is what the new generation of kids are up against. Most parents are now working two plus jobs to give their kids the "American Dream" (what does that even mean?). So, those crucial (sixty-one thousand) programming hours are now being substituted with various random programming: child care workers, TV shows, YouTube videos or hand held computers. Have you every stopped...and I mean really stopped... and thought deeply about what all of those outside influences are actually teaching your child?

One of the things I can say I did very well as a parent of four children, was sought out lots of advice. I read, (which was not easy for me as I used to hate to read) I don't know...maybe twenty to thirty books on parenting and went to many parenting classes, and I was raised in a very healthy family environment. My parents did a great job, they were engaged and stayed married their whole lives. I just knew though, in spite of that, I was not going to be able to do this without help. I knew anyone could become a parent, but very few know what they were doing. Do you realize you can't graduate high school without three years of math? To be a full time substitute teacher you need a four year bachelor's degree. To drive a Semi Truck, you need to go to driving school for three to four weeks. To be a Yoga instructor, you need two hundred hours of training. To remove a wart from a patient at the doctor's office, you need two additional years of schooling. To pull out a tooth from someone you barely just met, you need eight years of additional schooling but to have a child, you just have to... have sex. That's it! And you don't even need to be taught how to do that.

So, if you think to yourself, "I got this!" I don't even know what to say to that other than "WAKE UP"! Our kids deserve a shot at a somewhat normal life whether we had one or not. We all know the world around us is in no way normal but let's do our best to meet the basic core needs of our children. Those core needs are: Connection & Acceptance, Healthy Autonomy

& Performance, Reasonable Limits, Realistic Expectations and Spiritual Values and Community. You can find out more about those in the books that talk about schemas and life traps: "Reinventing Your Life" by Dr. Jeffrey Young and "Good Enough Parenting" by John and Karen Louis.

Now let's look at a few examples taken through the AOSED change process:

Example 1:

Tom is at a crossroads with his two kids. His wife has been telling him for years how his anger, bossiness and lack of patience is hurting his relationship with them. It is all he knows because that is how his father always treated him. The other night he went into his daughter's room to say goodnight and she would not speak to him. He went to bed that night and couldn't sleep. He knows he loves his kids but he does not know how to be close. He was never close with his father and, after laying there for hours thinking about why, he became aware that his father had never apologized for anything in his life, either to him or his mother.

PARENTING CHANGE PROCESS FORM

THE AWARENESS: (MUST BE PERSONAL AND DETAILED.)

I never apologize to my children. I see how this is hurting our relationship.

THE OBSTACLE: (MUST BE CLEARLY DETAILED AND DEFINED.)

I don't want to come across as weak. I want them to know who is boss. I think I am right all the time. My parents never apologized to me.

THE STRATEGY: (MUST BE THOUGHT OUT, DETAILED AND COMMITTED TO.)

Seek to understand the value of saying I am sorry. Practice saying this and meaning it. Put myself in their shoes.

WHAT IS THE NEW BELIEF YOU WANT TO HAVE?
(THIS IS A ROUGH DRAFT THOUGHT HERE. YOU WILL CLARIFY LATER IN THE PROCESS.)

I can apologize to my children and not feel weak.

Pros of This Choice	Cons of This Choice
They will forgive me	*Will need to learn to be humble*
We will be closer	
I can be better than my parents	
Will be close as they get older	
My wife will be amazed	
I will feel better about myself	
I can forgive myself	
Won't feel so bad about my parenting skills	
Lead by example	

(Take your time and write down as many Pros and Cons as you can think of! This helps solidify why this New Belief is valuable to you.)

WHAT THAT NEW STRATEGY LOOKS, SOUNDS AND FEELS LIKE.

Take a moment and close your eyes. Picture yourself already living out this New Belief.

Then describe in detail what you see, hear and feel.

Visual (I see...)

- *I see myself going into Sara's room and sitting on the bed to say I am sorry.*
- *I see myself sitting around the dinner table apologizing for raising my voice.*
- *I see Kyle asking me to take him to the park when I get home from work.*

145

Auditory (I hear...)

- *I hear Sara saying, "It's OK daddy, I forgive you."*
- *I hear my wife compliment me on how I handled that situation.*
- *I hear Kyle saying he is sorry to me for not obeying the first time.*

Kinesthetic (I feel...)

- *I feel peaceful. I feel light. I feel less burdened.*

THE EXECUTION: (MUST BE TIED TO YOUR STRATEGY AND PUT INTO MOTION IMMEDIATELY)

I will talk to my wife about this new change and get her input on how to start. Be aware of my tone of voice and try to listen before I blame or get mad. Ask the kids more questions first, before assuming the worst.

THE DESIRED RESULT: (YOUR NEW PERSONAL BELIEF STATEMENT)

I am able to easily apologize to my children from my heart.

WHOLE-BRAIN PROGRAMING: (This adds the New Belief to your subconscious. Before starting this final exercise, read though your whole change process form one more time.)

Get into a Whole-Brain Posture (sitting on a chair, legs and arms crossed).
Close your eyes and think about your new desired result belief statement.

"I am able to easily apologize to my children from my heart."

Concentrate on experiencing a mental, emotional or physical change in your mind and body about your New Belief statement as you repeat it over and over again silently.
After a few minutes you will feel a change in your thoughts, feelings or emotions.
Then open your eyes, uncross your body and Lock in the New Belief.

See appendix A in the back of this book for the detailed process of how to do the "Whole-Brain Programing" exercise.

Example 2:

Tammy is a single mom trying to raise three children on her own. She works full time and after work she is too tired to cook, so she gets takeout four to five times a week. She knows this is not healthy and she has seen how not only herself but the kids have put on a lot of excess weight. Her daughter has been complaining that the kids at school are teasing her and calling her fat. Tammy feels terrible and blames herself for this situation. She has decided to do something about it and comes up with a plan.

PARENTING CHANGE PROCESS FORM

THE AWARENESS: (MUST BE PERSONAL AND DETAILED.)

I am not taking care of the health of my children.

THE OBSTACLE: (MUST BE CLEARLY DETAILED AND DEFINED.)

I work too much and don't have time to cook. The kids have very busy schedules and we don't have time to sit down for dinner. It has not been a priority for me.

THE STRATEGY: (MUST BE THOUGHT OUT, DETAILED AND COMMITTED TO.)

I will talk to my boss about the possibility of taking a shorter lunch and leaving earlier. Have a talk with the kids about their schedules and if there is something they want to give up so we spend more time together. Make this a priority.

WHAT IS THE NEW BELIEF YOU WANT TO HAVE?
(THIS IS A ROUGH DRAFT THOUGHT HERE. YOU WILL CLARIFY LATER IN THE PROCESS.)

My children's wellbeing is my top priority.

Pros of This Choice	**Cons of This Choice**
We will all be less stressed	*Will take some work*
More time to spend together	*Have to reschedule*
I will be healthier myself	*More discipline*
Teach my children to prioritize	
Laugh and enjoy dinner together	
Get back to cooking which I love to do	
Time to get together with other families	
Hear more about what is going on in my kids' lives.	
Take family walks by the lake	
Teach the kids to cook	
My daughter will feel better about herself	

(Take your time and write down as many Pros and Cons as you can think of! This helps solidify why this New Belief is valuable to you.)

WHAT THAT NEW STRATEGY LOOKS, SOUNDS AND FEELS LIKE.

Take a moment and close your eyes. Picture yourself already living out this New Belief.
Then describe in detail what you see, hear and feel.

Visual (I see...)

- *I see myself sitting around the table sharing about my day with my children.*
- *I see the kids setting the table and working together.*
- *I see myself sitting in bed Sunday night planning the meals for next week.*

Auditory (I hear...)

- *I hear my daughter thanking me for spending so much time with her.*
- *I hear my boss telling me, "No Problem, your family time is very important."*
- *I hear nothing as we all sit on the couch having our quiet reading time together.*

148

Kinesthetic (I feel...)

- *I feel relaxed, I feel inspired, I feel empowered, I feel loved.*

THE EXECUTION: (MUST BE TIED TO YOUR STRATEGY AND PUT INTO MOTION IMMEDIATELY)

I will ask my boss to lunch tomorrow and discuss my options for getting off earlier. I will talk to the kids tonight about some changes we are all going to make to be together more. I will clean out the pantry this weekend and take the kids shopping after we plan the first week of meals together.

THE DESIRED RESULT: (YOUR NEW PERSONAL BELIEF STATEMENT)

I spend a lot of quality time with my children every week.

WHOLE-BRAIN PROGRAMING: (This adds the New Belief to your subconscious. Before starting this final exercise, read though your whole change process form one more time.)

Get into a Whole-Brain Posture (sitting on a chair, legs and arms crossed).
Close your eyes and think about your new desired result belief statement.

"I spend a lot of quality time with my children every week."

Concentrate on experiencing a mental, emotional or physical change in your mind and body about your New Belief statement as you repeat it over and over again silently.
After a few minutes you will feel a change in your thoughts, feelings or emotions.
Then open your eyes, uncross your body and Lock in the New Belief.

Being a parent is one of the greatest gifts from above. It means YOU have been chosen to have the honor of loving someone unconditionally. Someone who has your strengths and weaknesses. Someone who will bring out the things in your character you need to change, someone who will make you a better person by teaching you to deny yourself and put others first, (which is one of the greatest commands on earth). So work hard at being the best you can be. You may not be able to go backwards to fix all the mistakes you have made, but your Awareness will empower you to go forwards and become what your child needs, no matter what age they are. You are a parent for life, which means you have your whole life to get it right. Don't wait any longer.

P.S. Don't be afraid to use these change forms with your children.

For example: If your child comes home from school and tells you about a difficult situation with another kid or a teacher, share with them what has helped you make changes in your life and pull out the "Relationship" or Personal Growth" change form and teach them how to process like the example below:

RELATIONSHIP CHANGE PROCESS FORM

THE AWARENESS: (MUST BE PERSONAL AND DETAILED.)

My friend Jennifer is talking behind my back and spreading rumors.

THE OBSTACLE: (MUST BE CLEARLY DETAILED AND DEFINED.)

She is being mean to me. I want to cut her out of my life. She is telling lies.

THE STRATEGY: (MUST BE THOUGHT OUT, DETAILED AND COMMITTED TO.)

Ask her to come over to hang out. Share what I have heard and give her the opportunity to explain.

WHAT IS THE NEW BELIEF YOU WANT TO HAVE?
(THIS IS A ROUGH DRAFT THOUGHT HERE. YOU WILL CLARIFY LATER IN THE PROCESS.)

I will work this out and keep her as a friend.

150

Pros of This Choice	Cons of This Choice
Not so much drama	*I will have to be humble*
Stop the rumors	*I have to make the first move*
Have her apologize	
Find out if I did something	
to hurt her	
Keep a good friend	
Less stress at school	

(Take your time and write down as many Pros and Cons as you can think of! This helps solidify why this New Belief is valuable to you.)

WHAT THAT NEW STRATEGY LOOKS, SOUNDS AND FEELS LIKE.

Take a moment and close your eyes. Picture yourself already living out this New Belief.
Then describe in detail what you see, hear and feel.

Visual (I see...)

- *I see Jennifer and myself sitting on my bed talking.*
- *I see the both of us hugging.*
- *I see myself walking into school with Jennifer and we are laughing together.*

Auditory (I hear...)

- *I hear myself telling myself, "You did the right thing."*
- *I hear my mom telling me how proud she is of the way I handled that.*
- *I hear Jennifer apologize to me.*

Kinesthetic (I feel...)

- *I feel relieved, I feel happy, I feel encouraged.*

THE EXECUTION: (MUST BE TIED TO YOUR STRATEGY AND PUT INTO MOTION IMMEDIATELY)

Ask Jennifer today at lunch if she wants to come over tonight. If she says no I will keep asking her until she does.

THE DESIRED RESULT: (YOUR NEW PERSONAL BELIEF STATEMENT)

Jennifer and I work this out and we are still best friends.

WHOLE-BRAIN PROGRAMING: (This adds the New Belief to your subconscious. Before starting this final exercise, read though your whole change process form one more time.)

Get into a Whole-Brain Posture (sitting on a chair, legs and arms crossed).
Close your eyes and think about your new desired result belief statement.

"Jennifer and I work this out and we are still best friends."

Concentrate on experiencing a mental, emotional or physical change in your mind and body about your New Belief statement as you repeat it over and over again silently.
After a few minutes you will feel a change in your thoughts, feelings or emotions.
Then open your eyes, uncross your body and Lock in the New Belief.

Remember, no one runs off of their feeling and emotions more than your children. It is your responsibility to help them create healthy Beliefs. Imagine if you would help your child process a needed change of heart like the example above. Whereas some parents may just say to their daughter in this situation, "Honey, you don't need her as a friend, forget about her and move on. If someone does something like that to you, forget her!"

The changes you will make by taking the time to go through one of these exercises will amaze you. Feel free to download a set of "Change Process" forms that are already created for you to just fill in, they are available for download anytime at: **www.30MinuteChange.com**

The Ending

*"While some may fear the end is in sight. Others will see the
Journey as a never-ending circle in which one gets a
Second change the next time around."*

For some of you, this whole concept of changing
anything in your life in "30 Minutes" or less may just
seem too far-fetched. You may be thinking, "how
can something that I have tried for years to do, be this simple?"
Or, "I really don't see how this is going to work for me!" All I
can say to that is this: you have never tried to change something
in your life quite this way before, so that is not a fair
assessment, just a thought. And this process is not that simple!
Anyone can think about something in their life that needs to
change and then even start to do something about it, that's
simple! But actually, taking the time to go through this full
AOSED change process takes effort, training and intense
cognitive brain work. I believe a better question to ask yourself
is, "What will it cost me physically, emotionally, relationally,
spiritually or financially if I do not make the Desired Change?"

What if instead, you were able to just accept and surrender
to the fact that you do have total control to change your beliefs,
right now? That you will able to change, because you are now
actively thinking, doing and believing differently in your
present circumstances. This then allows your newly created

beliefs to overwrite your negative or limiting beliefs that were previous instilled by your less aware self with its vulnerable thoughts and emotions. That being said, this next powerful awareness is something I would like you to accept and begin to process going forward:

"I will not let just any random thought i.e. "emotion", become a belief, but rather I will program and allow only new "wanted" beliefs to become my new empowering thoughts."

This will help you overcome your "temporary" emotions by being able to draw from wanted and factual true beliefs.

Here is an example of this: Your spouse was rude to you this morning before work.

You love your spouse, you know they love you, you have been through so much together and you believe they will help you grow into a better person. Those are the facts and your true beliefs. But since your spouse was rude to you this morning and hurt your feelings, you now question (due to your emotions) if this is the right person for you, is it worth sticking with this relationship, I saw my parents go through this and it was ugly, I'm sure there is someone out there that would never treat me this way, blah, blah, blah! Those are only emotions! Not that they aren't true to you in that moment, but how much more empowered would you be if you could just stop those thoughts dead in their tracks, focus on your true beliefs and come to the simple conclusion that maybe your spouse was running late, they did not sleep well and maybe they are feeling lots of pressure at work. Instead, choose to send them a nice text and go on with your day in gratitude and living in the moment. By stopping the madness of your thoughts, you will have more control over your **emotions** and the effect they have on you in the moment than you realize!

Remember: **Your** thoughts are at the conscious level, but your beliefs are at the subconscious level. It is important to realize that many of those emotional rants are just memorized behaviors from past similar situations and your brain wants to attach them whenever it can.

You need to be very careful because your memorized emotions will **want** to keep you locked into your past. Once you realize you can unlock those unhealthy emotions by creating new healthy beliefs to override those programs, then your New Beliefs will cause you to behave differently and will give you New choices and experiences and these will in turn create New healthy emotions which will then build up your thoughts into creating even more New Beliefs. I call this the "Circle of Thought".

Understand this: By just setting aside 30 minutes, being alone in a quiet place, turning off all distractions (especially electronics) and **then** fully engaging your true thoughts on a wanted change and putting yourself though the whole AOSED change process...if you can do this, Holy Cow! Imagine the amount of focus and power you would give yourself in order to make the desired change. You first became self-Aware. You then took the time to think deeply about the Obstacles and their causes. You worked through a detailed Strategy, involving your senses in which you saw, heard and felt what it would be like experiencing that change. Which started the process of creating new circuits and connections in your brain. You took the time to develop the perfect Execution. You defined your New Belief statement about the Desired Change. Finally, you spent the time to meditate and lock in this new belief into your subconscious mind. Thus, every **action** creates a reaction!

Are you kidding me? **There** is no better formula for change out there. I know, I have tried most of them. If you still don't believe this will work for you, then this will be your first change to make.

- **Awareness:** I don't believe this process will work for me.
- **Obstacle:** I lack trust in new things or things I cannot control. Things that seem too easy for me, never are. I always start things but don't finish them.
- **Strategy:** I need help implementing this into my life. I must trust in something I don't fully understand. Finish one complete process.

The belief I want to have: "I completely trust and engage in the new 30 Minute Change process."
I see myself sitting on the couch going through the change process.
I see myself teaching my co-worker what I have learned.
I see me friends standing around asking me what's so different.
I hear my spouse tell me how much I have changed.
I hear the wind and the birds as I easily ride my bike around the lake.
I hear myself telling myself, "you can do anything you believe."
I feel excited about life. I feel energetic. I feel unstoppable. I feel

happy.

- **Execution:** I will sign up for the one time personal coaching session to help me better understand and execute the change process. After that, for the next three days, I will start and complete one new change process each morning before work. I will trust that the needed change will make an impact right away in my life.

- **Desired Result:** My New Belief statement is; *"I easily accept and encourage any needed change into my mind."*

Now sit and **reprogram** that into your subconscious brain and then Execute!

The 30-minute change process is something you learn to do with practice. It **gets** easier and easier with each change. Your New Beliefs will change the course of your life and open up opportunities you never thought existed. So now that you are done reading this book, you have a complete understanding of how to take yourself through the "AOSED" change process. Your only question moving forward is, "Will you, do it?"

In closing, I would like to suggest for you to invest in yourself if you have any doubt that you can do this on your own. What I have **experienced** since creating this process, is that the quickest and most effective way to learn how to take yourself through the process in 30 minutes or less, is done with the help of a "one-time", personal, one on one coaching session, done with an experienced coach over the phone. Your personal coach will help guide you through each step, by teaching you to ask yourself the right questions, helping you tap into the deeper thoughts about the needed change and then teaching you how to define your New Belief statement. This guarantees that by the time you're done with this 90-minute session, you will have learned how to complete one or more of your needed changes and you'll clearly understand afterwards how to develop your most effective New Belief statements. You will feel empowered and confident to use this process to change anything in your life going forward. And my hope is that you share what you have learned with others.

My final thoughts:

What I have learned as I get older is, the more I think I know, the less I actually know. **Things** that I thought were true years ago, sometimes change. That in most cases, simpler is actually better. And that God gave us two ears and one mouth for a reason. That being said, I hope you enjoyed what you have learned and that you will make the effort to take the steps and make at least one change. For many of you, it was just a reminder of what you already knew to be true, but may gave you a simplified interactive process to use going forward. For the rest of you, I believe it will set a new course for your future and how you make changes for the rest of your blessed life.

Just remember, everything is possible for the one who believes!

Thank you for spending this time with me and I hope you were able to spark some new Awareness.

Pat

Appendix A
Whole-Brain Posture

Sit comfortably in a chair crossing your feet at the ankles, right over left and then hold your arms out in front of you, palms facing outwards. Now cross **them** at the wrist, left over right with the thumbs facing down, clasp your hands together by interlocking your fingers and drop them in your lap and relax. (See below.)

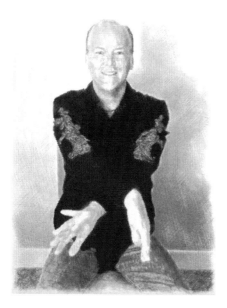
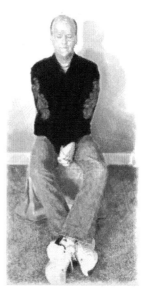

Place the tip of your tongue behind your upper front teeth. Then, while you're in this relaxed position, close your eyes and begin to repeat your New Belief Statement (Example: "I love and respect myself enough to only have healthy relationships.") over and over silently in your mind until you experience a mental, emotional or physical change in your mind and body about your New Belief. There may be other thoughts trying to distract you, just acknowledge and then release them like a fluffy cloud floating by. Remember to silently keep repeating your New Belief Statement.

After a few minutes you will feel a change in your thoughts, feelings or emotions. Once that happens, open your eyes, uncross your arms and legs. While still seated, lock in the New Belief by holding your hands in front of you in a prayer position for a few seconds while thanking yourself for accepting this New Belief of

_____!

That's it! The New Belief has been programmed into your subconscious. You just need to go and live out your New Belief by Executing your Strategy. Then, whenever your conscious mind repeats the old negative patterns about that belief, you just remind it of your newly created and subconsciously programmed New Belief statement.

References

- Lipton, B (2008). The Biology of Belief: *Unleashing the Power of Consciousness, Matter & Miracles.* New York, NY: Hay House Inc.

- Ridding M, et al. *Just 30 Minutes of Exercise Has Benefits for the Brain.* University of Adelaide. 2014.

- The Holy Bible, New International Version Grand Rapids: Zondervan House, 1984. Print.

- Williams, R (2004). Psych-K: *The Missing Peace IN Your Life.* Crestone, CO: The Myrddin Corporation

Coming In 2018

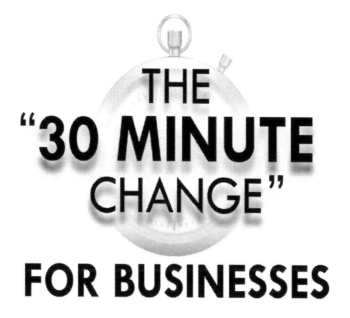

Learn how to use the "AOSED Change Process" to radically change and unify your company and its team members.

Made in the USA
San Bernardino, CA
06 July 2018